The Weight Loss Lifestyle

D0967227

Eric J. Belanger

The Weight Loss Lifestyle

Your Proven Starting Guide to Lose Weight and Get Healthier While Saving Time and Money

Eric J. Belanger, PA-C, MPAS

Eric J. Belanger

DEDICATION

This book is dedicated to my amazing wife, Elisha,
and the greatest sons a Dad could ever have -
Benjamin and Nathan.
And, to my remarkable patients.

Eric J. Belanger

TABLE OF CONTENTS

WHY I WROTE THIS BOOK

Thank you for taking the time to read this guide, I truly believe it will help you get started and provide helpful information. The reason I wrote this is simple – to provide people who wish to lose weight, get healthier, and feel better an easy, proven place to start.

Every day I work with patients who struggle with their health and weight. They have often tried every weight loss program and fad diet available and always end up at the same spot, sometimes even further behind than they were before.

For all of these patients I believe I have a helpful perspective and approach, however I am confronted with the situation of not having enough time in an office visit to tell them everything I want them to know to help them towards their goals.

This guide is the result of over a decade spent learning, researching, and experiencing all of the various perspectives and information concerning weight loss and becoming healthier. This isn't a fad diet or extreme fitness plan to be purchased and eventually forgotten. Using these fundamental principles with patients day after day has provided life-changing results for them.

My career as a physician assistant has allowed me to explore and trial ways to assist patients in drastically improving their lives. I've seen debilitating effects of chronic disease due to poor nutrition, sedentary lifestyles, and unhealthy habits.

As a health care provider, my education consists of a Bachelor of Science in Biomedical Sciences and a Master's Degree in Physician Assistant Studies. For over eleven years I've treated thousands upon thousands of patients in surgery and medical clinics. Also, as a busy professional, I myself have struggled with nutrition and getting enough activity into my day. Many of the recommendations are the ones I've used over the years to reach my own goals, so I know they work.

My hope for you is the best health you can possibly have for you and your family. I hope the words in these pages will encourage you to examine your life, find areas to improve, and get the results you want while improving your health and quality of life.

WHY YOU SHOULD READ THIS BOOK

You should read this book if you are currently overweight, obese, have overweight children or are overall unhappy with your health and wish to examine where things may have gone wrong and what easy, inexpensive action you can take to change direction.

You should read this book if these facts concern you:
• 70% - the percent of adult Americans classified as overweight in 2016.

• 39% - the percent of overweight adult Americans considered obese in 2016.

• 20% - the rate of obesity in our kids aged 12-19 years old.

• $190,000,000,000 – annual medical spending related to obesity and associated diseases in the US.

• 20% - the percent of our annual health care spending used to treat obesity and obesity-related diseases.

• $65,000,000,000 - spent on weight loss products in 2017 in the US. Yep, that's BILLIONS.

• 25% - the percent of Americans at least 65 years old with Type 2 diabetes in 2015.
Adapted from CDC.gov Fast Stats

The take away from this data is this: **if we have been spending enormous amounts of money and effort on weight loss however every year our weight is higher and our health is worse – maybe it's time to look at the big picture and spend a little bit of energy seeing where things are going wrong and put our energy into finding a better way and fixing the situation.**

This guide will help explain why a "big picture" approach is the best way to start improving your health, weight and quality of life.

CHAPTER 1

THE COMMON QUESTION!

The most common question patients ask me concerning improving their health or losing weight is: where do I start? Most patients have tried many different diets and various exercise programs but always come back to the same starting point.

After being in this cycle many times over the years, they are generally very frustrated, feel guilty, and intimidated about the idea of trying again. Every day we are bombarded by some new fad diet promising all kinds of dream-like results and outcomes. Maybe some celebrity has endorsed it and we think it might be worth a try. Maybe the six easy monthly payments or the low introductory rate for the membership seems reasonable. And, we buy it. We try it for a week or two, maybe even a month and then we're back to where we were. Except, we now have less in our bank account and a huge sense of guilt and low self-worth.

Ultimately, the fundamental principle behind this book is this: Achieving weight loss and getting healthier will happen if you really look at your lifestyle and replace unhealthy habits with healthier habits on a consistent basis. In my experience, restricting anything in your life generally makes a person obsess about what they can't have which essentially forces them to go get whatever it is they are trying to avoid. Also, we seem hardwired to need to spend our hard-earned money on programs, equipment, supplements and memberships when the data and our own experience clearly states we're fooling ourselves. We're not going to stick with it and deep in our hearts, we know it. Sure, maybe 10-15% can honestly stick with an added program or diet for a while but most of us can't. And again, we know it.

After working with patients day after day I've realized most people aren't really happy. They don't feel well, their lives aren't what they hoped they would be and they feel stuck. Tight finances and the stresses of modern life are wearing people out. We're tired, overwhelmed, and simply over it.

I believe I have found at least part of the answer to the issue of our overwhelmed modern lifestyle. It starts with more of a grassroots approach and the results have been astounding. Our jobs, families, friends and hobbies are missing one important thing: us. We're so busy anymore that we rarely get outside, most of our meals come out a window at the burger joint and our relationships are in the toilet. I believe the solution to most of these issues is improving the quality of food we eat, getting rid of the chemical and sugar-laden "healthy" food we've been sold, and getting active again in our homes, work places and our communities. How can adding more to our daily planners and seeing our family and friends less possibly improve our health? How can being stuck in an expensive, stuffy gym be more energizing than being outside or going for a walk with your children or a friend?

You'll likely notice nearly everything I recommend is completely opposite what the commercials and marketers try to sell you. You'll never hear me say if you're overweight that you need to run or start flipping over tires for your workout. And, you'll never hear me recommend spending more time away from your family and friends, or more time indoors, or more of your hard earned money on much of anything. This is because for most people it simply isn't the answer to the problem. In fact, maybe having gained a few pounds or being more stressed isn't actually the problem at all? Maybe the weight and poor health are actually only the symptoms of a bigger issue, which I think is the overwhelmed and convenience-based lifestyle we have allowed to control our lives. The lifestyle says we can't possibly walk a block to the store, we must drive. Our lifestyle says we must leave our families to go work out in an expensive gym instead of spending time with them. And, the lifestyle says we need to go broke doing it.

Well, I think it's wrong. I believe by reimagining how we want our lives to be, and making decisions based on our priorities, we can get back to healthier habits and feel well, without all the causes of being unhappy.

This, my friends, is where to start.

Habits

"First we form habits: then they form us.
Conquer your bad habits or they will conquer you."
~Robert Gilbert

Habits are the building blocks of your life. The habits you possess will take you in the direction you want to go. If you have unhealthy habits, you will be unhealthy. If you have healthy habits, you will likely be healthy. If your habit is to drink a 32 ounce soda several times daily, this habit will no doubt harm you. If, however, your habit is to take a daily walk, then this habit will improve your health. It's that simple.

We all have habits. We usually don't realize how many habits – good and bad – we actually have! For example, have you ever arrived at work safe and sound and realized you can't recall a single moment of your commute from home? Seriously, your commute could be five minutes or an hour long, but you honestly don't remember a moment? How many stoplights, stop signs and turns did you make and you don't remember a thing without really thinking about it? THIS is how powerful your habits are in your life. For better or worse habits allow us to be on autopilot most of our days.

Currently, you have habits which are most likely creating a situation leading to weight gain or poor health. These habits may include snacking, going out for lunch, drinking high calorie drinks or simply eating poor quality food. All of these simple habits combine to form the overall routine of your life. It is critical then for you to review your daily life routine for habits leading to your poor health.

The following poem describes the power of habits and the importance of being aware of them. Habits can be used to succeed or fail in life and in your health.

The Habit Poem

I am your constant companion.
I am your greatest helper or heaviest burden. I will push you onward or drag you down to failure.
I am completely at your command.
Half of the things you do you might as well turn them over to me and I will do them – quickly and correctly.
I am easily managed – you must be firm with me.
Show me exactly how you want something done and after a few lessons, I will do it automatically.
I am the servant of great people, and alas, of all failures as well.
Those who are great, I have made great.
Those who are failures, I have made failures.
I am not a machine though I work with the precision of a machine plus the intelligence of a person.
You may run me for profit or run me for ruin – it makes no difference to me.
Take me, train me, be firm with me, and
I will place the world at your feet.
Be easy with me and I will destroy you.
Who am I?
I am Habit.

~Author Unknown

Over time our habits can be modified, replaced, or eliminated all-together to help you reach our goals. The habits you'll use to lose weight and become healthier will be created exactly the same way as your old habits were created. Just as you have changed your habits in the past, you can easily incorporate new, healthier habits into your life.

Think about it this way: we have the HABIT of buying the same foods at the grocery store, we have the HABIT of driving everywhere to get things done, we have the HABIT of spending our evenings sitting in front of the TV or out for drinks at the bar, and we have the HABIT of paying good money for solutions which haven't worked.

A serious look at these habits is crucial to get to the heart of the matter. If we haven't stopped to consider we have a leak in our boat, how can we act to fix it before we all sink? Based on our increasing body weight, stress, illness, and overall unhappiness in life it's clear we are barely keeping our heads above water. It's clear we need to step back, think about the issues and only then work to address them. We simply must or soon we'll all be sunk.

Do It For The Kids!

Being a parent and caring for children is a very tough responsibility. It takes a lot of time, tons of energy and a plan. All too often we feed our children foods that aren't healthy out of convenience and sometimes necessity. I challenge us as a society to really consider and decide how important it is to feed our children healthy, nutritious meals. I hear many parents complain about the toxic school lunches fed to kids as part of the school lunch programs in the nation. My question is always this: why as a parent are you relying on their school to feed them and know what's best for them? Aren't you as the parent the ultimate authority on the foods your child eats? If you are a parent I encourage you to think about all the healthy habits presented in this book, both nutritional and activity habits, which you can incorporate into not only your life, but the lives of your children. The parent is the primary role model for children so when they observe their parents eating healthy and being physically active, this sets up a great, healthy family culture.

If you are able to start off your toddlers eating healthy, whole food you'll have a child who will likely be able to avoid a significant number of diseases and conditions in their lifetime due to the simple, yet powerful, habit of eating healthy. If your children are older, strive to change their eating habits and nutrition plan to more healthy foods. We all want the best for our own children and the children in our communities. Let's work together to keep them healthy and happy!

CHAPTER 2

YOUR NUTRITION PLAN!

*"We're the country that has more food to eat than any
other country in the world, and with more diets to keep us
from eating it."*
~Unknown

The goal of eating is to bring in essential nutrients
your body requires to stay healthy and survive. Most
people call the food you eat your diet, however these
days the word "diet" indicates you are generally
eating only certain foods while avoiding others in an
effort to lose weight or reach some other goal. The
words "diet" and "dieting" are very powerful words
and generally evoke a negative feeling. Often, these
words reflect past failures or bad results. To avoid
this, I ask you to refer to the foods you eat as either
your Nutrition or your Nutrition Plan. At first it
seems a bit strange to say however as you say it
several times, you'll notice it doesn't give you that
guilt-ridden, crummy feeling those other words gave

you. Referring to food as your Nutrition makes sense since the goal of eating is to provide your body with vital nutrients to keep it functioning at an optimal level.

Processed Food

> *"Processed foods not only extend the shelf life, but they extend the waistline as well."*
> ~Karen Sessions

Human food has looked and tasted pretty much the same for several hundred thousand years. Only recently over the past 50-75 years has our food become significantly altered, or processed, to remove certain components and to add others in. Surprisingly, many people believe our increasing weight and poor health trend has been occurring over hundreds, if not thousands of years. This couldn't be more wrong. Again, the worsening of our health as a society and increased weight has only been occurring for less than about 50 years. A review of the data indicates this situation is relatively new and we're only now realizing what is wrong and what to do about it.

As a society, we've been led to believe foods labeled with healthy-sounding words like "Fat Free, Low Fat, Reduced Fat, Light and Lite" are healthy but they are actually the least healthy foods you could possibly buy. These foods were created by food industry marketing experts and made to appear to be the healthier option compared to the original food since the original dietary guidelines made fats the enemy. The crazy part is these foods are generally much more expensive even though they are actually less healthy. Research proves that fat is actually less dangerous in nearly every scenario than the added sugar in processed foods. The high intake of carbohydrates is the main culprit causing our current obesity epidemic and increasing rates of pre-diabetes and Type 2 diabetes.

Whenever you read the words "processed" or "refined," you should immediately think, "Nutrients removed, Chemicals added."

For example, think about a strawberry which has great fiber, taste, and no chemical additives. The ingredient list for a strawberry is: strawberry.

Now, think about a strawberry fruit product. Here is the ingredient list:

Grapes From Concentrate, Sugar, Maltodextrin, Corn Syrup, Pears From Concentrate, Partially Hydrogenated Cottonseed Oil, Carrageenan, Citric Acid, Acetylated Mono and Diglycerides, Sodium Citrate, Malic Acid, Xanthan Gum, Vitamin C (Ascorbic Acid), Locust Bean Gum, Natural Flavor, Potassium Citrate, Color (Yellow 5, Red 40, Blue 1).

See what I mean? There isn't even any strawberry in this strawberry fruit product! It's ridiculous! And, they actually added in a synthetic form of vitamin C just to make it sound healthy. You can guarantee on the exciting, colorful label there is a banner saying "Great source of Vitamin C!" Do you know what an even better source of vitamin C is? An actual strawberry! Mind blown.

For some reason we are completely fine with being lied to about the contents of our food. But, what if you paid a lot of money for a high quality diamond, only to find out it is worthless cubic zirconia? Why aren't we as humans just as upset at a company charging us a high price for a synthetic chemical bomb that is supposed to be healthy food? We need to honestly think about this as a society. They won't sell it if we don't buy it but unfortunately things are looking pretty good for them, and not so good for us.

If your food doesn't spoil within a week or two of buying it, it isn't food, it's a chemistry experiment.

Think about it another way - for thousands upon thousands of years, humans have lived on meat, vegetables, nuts and fruit. Our remarkable bodies are optimized to extract nutrients including vitamins and minerals from these sources. We don't need expensive and complicated replacements. Nature has figured it all out already. It's only during the past 50 years of humans getting involved that we've managed to screw it all up. It is your personal responsibility to decide which type of food you think will result in your body being healthier, feeling better and functioning at its best: real food or "synthetic" food? It really is that simple. The decision is even easier if you're a parent since we want the absolute best for our children and prefer to feed our children the healthiest food we can afford. So I ask; why shouldn't you have the best nutrition, too? Think about it.

When I recommend removing certain foods or food products from their nutrition plan, the most common question people immediately ask me is, "what should I replace it with?" My answer is easy; you should simply replace it with more of the other healthy foods you are currently eating or plan on eating. Just because you remove or avoid something doesn't mean it has to be exactly replaced with a specific category or type of food.

People always need strict answers to what to do or not to do, however, they rarely actually follow the answer provided. This is why I provide very clear recommendations on how to eat healthier and get more active however I don't tell you exactly what to do or not do simply because I've found the people who have the best success are the ones who really take a good look at their lives, figure out what they personally need to change, and then actually change it so it works for them. It's the same problem for everyone but a different solution for each one.

Dietary Guidelines

In the late 1970's and early 1980's, the original dietary guidelines were published in the United States which ultimately led to the original food pyramid. Using flawed data, Americans were advised to avoid fats and eat up to 65% carbohydrates. Carbohydrates, or carbs, are various forms of simple sugars, complex chains of sugars called complex carbohydrates, and fiber. Simple carbs are any of the various forms of sugar including table sugar, high fructose corn syrup and other simple sugars. Complex carbohydrates are foods such as rice, flour, beans, whole wheat, legumes, potatoes and vegetables. The original guidelines indicated fats were the enemy while carbohydrates, low fat processed foods, and whole grains were deemed the healthiest and best foods to eat. We now know this is completely backwards. In fact, it's the single reason for the skyrocketing number of overweight and obese Americans and also the increasing rate of pre-diabetes and Type 2 diabetes in our society. Unfortunately, this high carbohydrate and convenience–based, unhealthy way of eating has spread over most of the globe and continues to spread rapidly.

I could spend hours discussing the complexities and errors in the original dietary guidelines and all of the various undercurrents of subsidies, lobbyists and influencers. To save you time you'll never get back, I've elected to let it go and move on. If you're interested, simply go online and you'll find more than you ever wanted to know.

Avoid Grains

A majority of American food contains grains which is a huge problem. Grains and flour cause a huge blood sugar and insulin spike after eating them which is why you end up being hungry again about an hour after you eat an entire bowl of oatmeal in the morning. The hormone insulin tells your body store fat if possible and makes you hungry again. I recommend completely avoiding the bakery section at the grocery store so you can avoid buying breads, baked goods and especially whole grain products. Even though "whole grain" sounds healthy, it's a metabolism bomb. Whole grain, oatmeal, rice and granola have been sold to Americans as a healthy alternative to any food containing fat but they are not the better option. Look at any processed food and you'll usually find some kind of flour, corn additive or wheat-based additive. As a society we're starting to see a large increase in sensitivities to various grains, especially wheat and gluten. Several years ago I found out I had celiac disease, the immune system disorder which causes the digestive system to essentially go into nuclear crisis mode when gluten or wheat has been consumed. At first I was devastated since I couldn't have donuts, beer and breads. After a month or so of avoiding wheat products and eating more whole foods, I realized I felt incredible and had tons of energy! This is actually a common experience for many people who adhere to low/no grain nutrition plans for one reason or another. Many people experience bloating, gas, diarrhea and constipation after eating grain-filled products and don't even realize it is the grain causing the issue. I know a lot of beer drinking, good old boys who go for decades not realizing why they have explosive diarrhea after a night of drinking beer. Again, human beings DO NOT need to consume carbohydrates or whole grain to survive. The high consumption of grain-based food and carbohydrates has created a disaster for our health due to the increase in our weight and the incidence of pre-diabetes and Type 2 diabetes. I recommend avoiding these as much as you can.

Please Note: The use of the word "diabetic" in this guide refers specifically to TYPE 2 diabetes. Type 1 diabetes has a completely different cause and is NOT the type of diabetes being discussed or referred to in this guide in any way.

CHAPTER 3

PRE-DIABETES AND TYPE 2 DIABETES!

Please do not skip this chapter thinking it doesn't apply to you! Nearly HALF of all Americans are pre-diabetic or have Type 2 diabetes! Yes, this seems like a lot of people, because it is. Most people who are pre-diabetic have not been diagnosed yet so they have NO IDEA they are already headed down this road! The numbers show YOU are likely one of them and this information likely applies to you or a family member. You may have pre-diabetes and not even know it. Therefore, please don't skip this chapter as it may have everything to do with you and might completely change the course of your health and life!

As the food industry started creating more processed foods we saw the rate of Type 2 diabetes start to rise. Then, Americans were told not to eat fat and almost overnight there were thousands of processed foods on the shelves labeled "Lite, Low Fat, Reduced Fat, and Fat Free." Why is this a problem?

Because when the fat was removed, it was replaced by cheap carbohydrates, lots of carbohydrates. Currently, our country feeds itself primarily using carbohydrates. This is a big problem, and only getting bigger. As stated earlier, the overconsumption of carbohydrates is primarily responsible for pre-diabetes and Type 2 diabetes. So, these conditions are really dietary conditions and primarily due to the foods we eat on a consistent basis, year after year.

A vast majority of our foods are either carbohydrate-based like breads, pastas, candy and soda or they have sugars and other forms of carbohydrates added to them. Don't believe me? Look at the ingredients list of snack foods, prepared foods, freezer meals, or other processed foods which have these healthy-looking labels. Did you know there are over 50 different names for sugar added to processed foods? These have names like sugar, high fructose corn syrup, cane sugar, maltose, malt, etc. The point is this: sugars and other carbohydrates are the worst possible addition to pretty much any food and it's killing us. Currently, 80% of our foods have a form of sugar added to it.

There are no essential carbohydrates or sugars humans need in order to survive however our bodies do require essential fatty acids from fats and amino acids from protein. Our remarkable human metabolism allows us to eat essentially anything and convert it to glucose for our brain to use. Therefore, if we don't even need to eat carbohydrates to survive but we end up eating enormous amounts of carbohydrates nearly every day, you can expect it's going to be an issue, and it is. Long term consumption of high amounts of carbohydrate is toxic to your body.

Think of gaining weight due to a high intake of sugar and other carbohydrates like this: let's say you have a sports car with a full tank of premium gasoline and even though you don't need to, you pick up pieces of heavy firewood and load them into the back of the sports car as you drive around all day long. You think "I might need this source of energy later so I'll store it up." But since you already have a full tank of higher efficiency premium fuel and the firewood isn't even needed, all it ends up doing is adding a lot of extra weight to your sports car. This ends up decreasing its fuel efficiency and prematurely wearing out the various important parts like engine, suspension, tires, and ultimately doesn't end up being an advantage or useful at all. In fact, it ends up being a significant disadvantage since your once agile, sleek sports car is now like a slow, tired, dump truck packed full of heavy, inefficient fuel it doesn't even need.

This is what happens to our bodies when we consume high amounts of carbohydrates over the years and end up storing them as extra weight. Unfortunately, the added weight to our "vehicle" also wears out our parts; except our parts are our hearts, lungs, hips, knees, backs, and everything else. Also, our parts can't be simply replaced at the local repair shop when they prematurely wear out due to the extra wear and tear. When they're damaged, they're damaged. Best to empty out the extra firewood and get your vehicle back to being sporty and agile to prevent a significant number of visits to your local "body shop" which is well-equipped with expensive hospital beds, operating rooms and dialysis machines!

However, it is important to note a person can be pre-diabetic or a Type 2 diabetic and not be considered overweight or obese at all. In fact, in my opinion, this is likely the single reason many people are not aware they are pre-diabetic or Type 2 diabetic since most people believe they have to be overweight or obese to have these conditions. This is simply not true as I have many patients who are not overweight or obese and have pre-diabetes and Type 2 diabetes. For this reason, I recommend an annual checkup with your primary care provider for appropriate preventative care and annual blood work.

Many people don't understand the real issue when they are told they have insulin resistance, pre-diabetes, or Type 2 diabetes. What you need to understand is the body is metabolically able to deal with the high amounts of consumed carbohydrates for quite a while but eventually it becomes overwhelmed and it just can't keep up. The result is pre-diabetes and eventually, Type 2 diabetes.

Here is a very basic analogy for Type 2 diabetes: imagine a house in the middle of the freezing arctic with subzero temperatures outside. To heat this house there is a furnace which has a set point of 70 degrees. Currently, the home is warm and comfortable with everything running smoothly. Now imagine that some freezing arctic air starts leaking into the home. The air temperature drops below 70 degrees and the furnace kicks on to warm the house back up to its set point. Now, let's imagine the leak gets worse and blows in even more cold air into the house. Now the furnace has to work even harder to keep the temperature at the 70 degree set point. And, for a while, the furnace is able to keep up and maintain the temperature in the home pretty close to the set point as long as it runs constantly. However, over the years as more and more cold air comes into the house, the furnace isn't able to keep up and the cold air fills the home since the furnace isn't able to pump out enough warm air.

In our bodies, the pancreas is responsible for maintaining our blood sugar set point by secreting insulin to deal with elevated blood sugar. However, when a person constantly consumes high levels of carbohydrates (cold air), the pancreas (furnace) has to work overtime to try and keep up with the onslaught of extra sugar in the blood and to keep the circulating blood sugar at the natural set point. Similar to the furnace, the pancreas simply can't keep this up forever and the blood sugars start to consistently exceed the natural set point. This is essentially pre-diabetes.

At this point, if the carbohydrate intake is reduced to correct the situation, then the pancreas is able to manage this and things might be able to return back to normal. However, if consumption of high amounts of carbohydrates continues long term, then various medications and eventually insulins will be needed to reduce the blood sugar and provide enough insulin to deal with the high levels of carbohydrates, this is Type 2 diabetes.

So, to avoid burning out the pancreas like an overworked furnace, keeping the carbohydrate intake low and allowing your body to maintain its natural set point is the key to overall health and can prevent you from developing pre-diabetes and Type 2 diabetes.

Currently, about 48% of adult Americans are either insulin resistant or have Type 2 diabetes.

This is 1 in 2 of us and it's insane. So, if we know eating high amounts of carbohydrates is toxic then why do the current dietary guidelines still recommend around half of our daily nutrition be from carbohydrates? It seems crazy, because it is.

Also, most patients I see in clinic believe these conditions are permanent and progressive once they have been diagnosed as pre-diabetic and Type 2 diabetic. This is completely false. Since these conditions are primarily due to eating moderate to high amounts of carbohydrate, then significantly limiting or completely avoiding carbohydrates should reverse the process, which it does. Again, mild blown.

Here's another analogy: let's say you encounter a person in a bar who is drunk. What caused them to become drunk? Did the glass bottle do it? The bar? Their metabolism? Their family history? Their bone structure? Their work? Nope, none of these caused them to become drunk. They became drunk because they consumed a moderate to high amount of alcohol. That's it. So what simple advice would you give someone who doesn't want to get drunk? Your common sense advice would be: don't consume moderate to high amounts of alcohol. Following this logic then you should also tell a person who doesn't want to become pre-diabetic or Type 2 diabetic to avoid moderate to high levels of carbohydrates, right? Right. And it works. It's the exact same cause and effect scenario. If you consume the cause, then you'll develop the effect.

And another analogy: the toxic level of carbohydrates in your body when you are insulin resistant, pre-diabetic or Type 2 diabetes is similar to being exposed to something like poison ivy. By exposing your body to poison ivy (carbs), your body reacts with a rash (chronic, high blood sugars) which requires you to use medication (metformin, insulins, etc.) to treat the rash as long as the rash is present. So, wouldn't it make more sense to simply remove the poison ivy (carbs) from our body so the rash (chronic, high blood sugars) goes away and we no longer need daily rash medications (metformin, insulins, etc.)? It seems pretty simple to me, because it really is.

If you reduce the amount of carbohydrates you eat then these conditions will likely significantly improve, completely resolve, or at the very least, not progress and become worse. When a Type 2 diabetic starts a low/no carb nutrition plan, they are removing the carbohydrates which then reduces the amount of medication they need to use since their blood sugars are consistently lower. Type 2 diabetes medications function to reduce the level of blood sugar however they don't prevent the sugar in the blood from being elevated in the first place. This is the main issue. So with pre-diabetes and Type 2 diabetes medications, they don't actually treat the cause which is moderate to high carbohydrate consumption, they treat the effects which are chronically high levels of blood sugar.

This is why there is nothing to "cure" with pre-diabetes or Type 2 diabetes. The way to get rid of these conditions is to simply stop consuming the cause which is giving you the effect. If you want to avoid becoming drunk, then avoid moderate to high amounts of alcohol. If you want to avoid becoming pre-diabetic or Type 2 diabetic, then stop eating moderate to high amounts of carbohydrates. So when I indicate you can "reverse" pre-diabetes and Type 2 diabetes, this means you can reverse the situation which is causing you to have pre-diabetes and Type 2 diabetes, thereby lowering your blood sugars and possibly not having these conditions in the future.

Finally, by saying pre-diabetes and Type 2 diabetes is reversible or can be improved, I'm not saying the damage from these conditions can be simply returned to normal or made perfectly healthy again. The damage is usually permanent however doing anything you can to slow or reverse the progression of pre-diabetes and Type 2 diabetes is absolutely worth your time and effort. Also, many Type 2 diabetics have been on moderate to high levels of insulin medications for many years or even decades. When a person has been on insulins for this long it is not something which can be modified or reversed as easily, but it can be done. In this situation, however, reducing or eliminating the consumption of carbohydrates under the care of their primary care provider or diabetes specialist is completely worth looking into and may prevent further damage to their body.

Please note: If you have been diagnosed with Type 2 diabetes and take medications for this, check with your health care provider before adopting a low/no carb nutrition plan as all of your current medications are specifically titrated to your usual carb intake. Suddenly reducing your carb intake can throw your blood sugars and insulin response into chaos. However, being aware of the carbs you eat and slowly limiting these foods will reduce your blood sugars and your values will trend lower, which is a good thing.

Chronic, elevated blood sugar damages all of the smallest blood vessels in the human body. Can you guess where the smallest vessels are found and which diseases they can cause when they're damaged? These tiny vessels are found in the heart (heart attack), brain (stroke), kidneys (high blood pressure, dialysis), genitals (erectile dysfunction), eyes (blindness), nerves (nerve damage and burning), hands and feet (cold, poor blood flow). Do you happen to know any friends or family members who might have one or several of these conditions? I thought so...

Damaging Effects of Insulin Resistance, Pre-diabetes and Type 2 Diabetes:

• **Heart Damage** – A diabetic is 2-3 times more likely to die of heart attack or stroke. These are the leading causes of death in diabetics. Chronic, elevated blood sugars are toxic to the blood vessels, which supply oxygen and nutrients to the heart, and also increase your blood pressure. Both of which is the 1-2 punch to your heart and brain. The phrase "what could possibly go wrong?" applies here.

• **High Cholesterol** - Eating a lot of carbohydrates also increases the triglycerides in your blood which increases your total cholesterol and greatly increases your chance for artery-clogging plaque formation. Do you know the fastest way to improve your cholesterol numbers? Reduce your carbohydrate consumption and your triglycerides will probably drop like a rock! So, isn't it interesting that decreasing consumption of sugars and carbohydrates decreases your cholesterol and decreases your risk of heart disease? Feel free to go online and search for more information on this as it's eye-opening.

• **Kidney Damage** –Your kidneys filter blood. Diabetic nephropathy is the result of damage to your kidneys from chronically elevated blood sugars. Think of it like this: your kidneys act like noodle strainers to filter out the waste water from our blood. When a person has diabetic kidney damage, it's as if they have small carbohydrate noodles clogging the drain holes. As more damage occurs and more holes become clogged, the waste water can't filter through the kidney and their blood becomes increasingly toxic. If you don't want a "No Expense Paid Trip to Dialysis Three Times a Week," then lower your carbohydrate intake and protect your kidneys.

• **Eye Damage** – Diabetic eye damage causes loss of vision and puts you at higher risk of cataracts and glaucoma. There are some various treatments which can help, however, once you lose your vision, you can NEVER get it back. One of the saddest situations to deal with in healthcare is treating someone who is losing or has lost their vision due to completely preventable causes. Their level of regret is palpable and there is nothing anyone can do about it.

• **Diabetic Neuropathy** – Your entire body depends on a wiring system which uses nerves to take electrical signals to and from every part of your body in order to function correctly. Chronic, elevated blood sugar causes these nerves, especially the smallest ones, to become damaged (seeing a pattern yet?). People with diabetic neuropathy literally suffer day and night with burning, stinging and the feeling like their hands and feet are on fire. This is an incredibly common condition in the United States and requires costly medical care. The nerve damage also causes lack of sensation or numbness which causes sufferers to lose their ability to sense damage or injury to their skin. This causes people with poorly controlled diabetes to require surgical amputation of toes, feet, legs and hands due to chronic diabetic ulcers. It's essentially "whittling" away body parts every several weeks to months as the toxic sugar levels cause tissue death. I was involved in these procedures for many years as an orthopedic surgery physician assistant. I'll never forget the awkward irony when a patient had literally snuck a donut into the surgical suite to eat while we were amputating his toes. He was completely unable to mentally link the habit of eating sugary, carbohydrate-rich foods and losing his limbs. Since he had completely lost feeling in his feet he figured he could stay awake during the amputation and eat his donut. As I think about it now, maybe he had actually made the connection but felt it was too late. Either way, please avoid the scalpel by reducing your carbohydrate intake, lowering your blood sugars and preventing this horrific, stomach-churning scene.

• **Stomach Gastroparesis** – This occurs when the nerves controlling your stomach are damaged and your stomach is not able to move food through which causes delayed emptying. This condition can result in heartburn, reflux, bloating, stomach spasms and nausea.

In summary, if you do nothing else for yourself regarding improving your nutrition, do this: Significantly decrease the amount of carbohydrates and processed foods you eat. Strive to eat fresh, whole foods in their original form and avoid "foods" packaged in cardboard, plastic, or metal. Eat fresh and avoid packaged "food" like your life depends on it, because it does.

CHAPTER 4

WHERE TO FIND NUTRITION!

In my experience with patients who are trying to lose weight and become healthier, I've noticed about 80% of the solution is simply modifying the foods they eat and only about 20% is changing their physical activity. So, if you want to make progress and have some quick success, simply educating yourself about which foods to eat and which to generally avoid will start you in the right direction. There are hundreds of ways to get calories out, there is only one way to get them in.

Eat Whole Food

> *"Don't eat anything your great-great grandmother wouldn't recognize as food."*
> ~Michael Pollan

Whole food is best defined as food that has not been processed or refined and is in its original form, free from additives or other artificial substances. Whole food should comprise a large amount of the food you eat on a daily basis. Whole food is the complete opposite of processed food as it contains the highest density of nutrients including vitamin, minerals, fiber, proteins and healthy fats. By striving to eat foods in their original, unprocessed form you have the best chance of providing your body with everything it needs to function at the highest level. You can eat very healthy and relatively inexpensively by only buying foods in their original form with no processing and minimal packaging. Foods in their whole food forms are found along the perimeter of the grocery store. These foods include fruits and vegetables, meats and seafood, dairy, and eggs.

Perimeter Shopping

If you imagine your local grocery store, you will realize all of the fresh foods such as fruits and vegetables, meat and seafood, dairy and eggs are all along the outside walls, or the perimeter, of the store. In the center of the store are the aisles which contain mostly highly processed, refined and packaged foods. Grocery stores have an easier time displaying, cooling, watering and stocking fresh foods along the perimeter of the store compared to the rigid aisle shelves. Processed foods come in cans and boxes which are easier to stack on shelves. Vegetables and fruits don't stack very well so they require different displays. Eventually the fresh food will spoil if it isn't purchased. If a majority of the foods you buy at the grocery store could eventually spoil or go bad, then you're on the right track.

In the aisles of the grocery store on the shelves you'll find the processed and packaged foods which are designed to sit on the shelves for months or even years until they are purchased. These processed foods contain dyes, fillers, sugar, preservatives and other chemicals designed to improve the appearance and taste of food so you'll want to buy it even though your animal instinct says, "Danger! This looks like poison!"

Just like the "food products" in the aisles, the products in the bakery section and hot food case in the grocery store are essentially the recently created versions of the processed aisle foods. The chemical bombs including store brand cookies, muffins, cakes as well as the hot food case with "food products" like deep fat fried burritos, cheese sticks and corndogs should be avoided at all costs.

Your goal should be to maximize your shopping time along the perimeter of the store in order to buy fresh foods and minimize time in the aisles where the processed foods are located.

> *"Never be afraid to do something new.*
> *Remember, amateurs built the ark;*
> *professionals built the Titanic."*
> ~Anonymous

If you don't bring processed food products into your home then you won't be able to eat them, which reduces your exposure of chemical-filled foods and added forms of sugar. Try and avoid shopping in the aisles at the grocery store as much as possible. You'll eat significantly healthier if your habit is to shop around the perimeter of the store. Think about this next time you go to your favorite grocery store. It'll become remarkably obvious how simple this one simple trick can drastically improve your nutrition. However, I do have one question, why are most of the grocery stores in the United States oriented for shoppers to shop in a counter-clockwise direction? Chew on that!

When it comes to your nutrition, I want you to think about what you are really shopping for when you're in the store. You're shopping for nutrients, as many as you can buy for as little cost as possible. Most people buy the same 20-25 foods each week out of habit whether for ourselves or for the entire family. An easy way to eat much healthier is to replace some less healthy food options with healthier, natural, whole foods.   For example, instead of buying sweetened apple juice, buy a bag of apples instead. If you simply modify your weekly shopping list to include healthier, fresh foods, then your habit will be to buy this new, healthier set of foods automatically without any more life-sucking decisions or the exhausting use of willpower.   The decisions have already been made and there is no reason to reinvent the wheel on a weekly basis.   Why not make losing weight and getting healthier as easy, inexpensive and effortless as possible?

Perimeter Stop #1: Vegetables and Fruits

The one undisputed element of any healthy eating plan is to use vegetables and fruits as a large percentage of your daily nutrition intake.   These foods have tons of nutrients, fiber, water, and are easily digested.   I recommend trying to eat a wide variety of vegetables and fruits in as close to their original form as possible.   There are hundreds of different vegetables and fruits available; all have different vitamin and mineral contents.   Try not to get focused on certain nutrient profiles or benefits of one individual food.

The easiest and most effective way to shop for vegetables and fruits is to have as many colors in your shopping cart as possible. If you follow this one rule, there are essentially no further decisions that need to be made or thought that needs to go into shopping for fruits and vegetables. Think: lots of colors, in their original form, and then move on.

Here are some examples of color groups:

Red options include: apples, peppers, cabbage, onions, tomatoes, beets, radishes, pears, strawberries, raspberries, etc.

Yellow options include: peppers, corn, bananas, summer squash, beets, and pears, etc.

Orange options include: carrots, oranges, cantaloupe, grapefruit, pumpkin, squash, mangoes, and peaches, etc.

Green options include: avocado, apples, spinach, lettuce, green beans, kale, broccoli, cucumber, asparagus, and arugula, etc.

These are only general color examples of various vegetables and fruits. Many of these have multiple colors and textures. Remember, especially for fruits, it's best to eat them in their whole form including the skin if possible so you don't get a big blood sugar spike from eating just the juice. Again, eating the fiber also helps you feel full which is important to reducing the amount of food eaten in a day. Fiber is the reason we would struggle to eat an entire five dollar bag of carrots in a week but can eat an entire five dollar bag of potato chips in about ten minutes! Well, at least I can!

Vegetables are easy to prepare which makes them a great part of any meal even if you don't know how to cook very well. Strive to buy vegetables in their freshest form as much as you can. Avoid canned vegetables if possible as these are slowly having their nutrients leached out into the canned water or syrup. Frozen, sliced vegetables are a great alternative to eating fresh vegetables if necessary. I recommend going to the freezer section of the grocery store and buying the store brand or generic brand of vegetables since these usually only contain the sliced vegetable and some water. Avoid the seasoned or processed forms of vegetables to avoid added preservatives and fillers. Frozen vegetables store well and can be opened and sealed up several times which makes them much more convenient and reduces food waste. Simply steam or microwave them and they're ready to go.

A great lunch prep trick is to put some frozen, sliced veggies such as broccoli, cauliflower, and carrots into your Bento-style lunch box and they will stay nearly frozen until lunch time. Simply warm up your lunch in the microwave and they are ready to enjoy!

Easy Health Trick: My family usually has a cutting board set up on our counter so when we want a snack we simply reach into the produce drawer of our refrigerator and slice up veggies or fruit instead of reaching into the freezer for ice cream. Our children know to look at the cutting board first and only if there is nothing sliced up do they look in the pantry. It is actually pretty amazing how much more fresh vegetables and fruit we eat as a family using this one trick. Kids and adults on the run easily grab slices of cucumber and don't even question it! It's easy to slice up some produce if the cutting board is out; it usually takes a bit of work to get a bowl of ice cream ready to eat!

Many patients ask my opinion about fruit since it is sweet and is sugary. My rule is this: only eat fruit if you have to chew it. In other words, eat the fruit in its natural form such as an apple, slices of orange or berries as the whole fruit. Don't drink fruit juice as it is complete garbage. Fruit juice is merely the pure sugar form of fruit with all of the fiber removed and sugar likely added to improve the taste and help it last longer. Honestly, look at the ingredient label of your favorite orange or apple juice. Sure, fruit juice is an ingredient but what about all of the other ingredients which have been added in? It is garbage; all of it. I don't care if the juice is "High in Calcium" or "Pulp Added," in that case it is healthy-sounding garbage. Even if your juice doesn't have additives it still spikes your blood sugar and insulin which immediately leaves your body to believe that it needs to store all of the extra "juice" calories as fat. Your body and checking account will thank you when you buy a bag of apples and oranges which will last a week or two compared to a half gallon of fruit juice that lasts two days.

Perimeter Stop #2: Protein and Fats

The other two important macronutrients are proteins and fats. It's important to consume enough protein and fats for your body to function properly. However, there is a significant amount of debate regarding the best amount of protein and fats, and what types or sources of protein and fats, a person should consume in a day. A person can essentially find research to back any up any opinion or point of view.

As perimeter foods, it's important to have a simple list of the best protein and fat sources to add to your nutrition plan. Since I think a big picture view for your nutrition is the easiest and best, I recommend obtaining protein and some fat from eggs, chicken, beef, pork, and fish as well as beans, peas, lentils, nuts and tofu.

If you don't mind eating animals and their byproducts, then eat eggs and lean meat sources. If you wish to avoid animal sources for your proteins and fats, then eat the beans, peas, lentils and tofu. See how easy that was? You have every right as a human being to decide what the best option is for you and your family. Therefore, choose what works best for you and run with it!

Which oils to include in your nutrition plan is something to consider as well. I recommend using pure avocado, olive, coconut, sesame, and grape seed oils. These can and should be used in cooking prepared dishes and some can be drizzled on salads as dressings instead of processed, chemical and sugar-filled dressings. Also, a little butter goes a long way and allows you to avoid butter substitutes which are processed and generally regarded as no healthier in the big picture.

Perimeter Stop #3: Dairy

Dairy products are another perimeter food worth deciding whether or not to add to your nutrition plan. The risks and benefits of dairy products can be a "cow-sized" source of debate when it comes to the subject of healthy eating. That said, some dairy products including skim milk and cheese can be great sources of protein and fat.

If you consider the big picture, what is mammal milk, like cow and goat, designed to do? It is used to fatten a baby cow or goat up as fast as possible which improves its chance for survival. So, is this milk ultimately good or bad for humans? You can easily find research supporting both sides. The original dietary guidelines included dairy products as a critical aspect of good nutrition. However, many meats, vegetables, fruits and nuts are also excellent sources of calcium including salmon, almonds, kale, beans, broccoli, and figs. So, maybe humans don't need to be consuming as much dairy as was previously recommended? My big picture approach is this: it seems appropriate and reasonable to have some skim or 2% milk occasionally and enjoy cheeses a bit more often. However, if you choose to limit your dairy intake this is likely reasonable as well, especially if you are lactose intolerant or get stomach issues due to dairy products.

Consider the source: I recommend paying attention to where your meats, dairy products and eggs come from. There are many options available however I recommend buying the highest quality meats, eggs and dairy you can afford from the healthiest sources possible to avoid the chemicals and antibiotics the animals may have been exposed to.

Consuming protein and fats from the listed sources you prefer on a daily basis will supply the nutrients your body needs and will complement your intake of fresh vegetables and fruits. The goal is to get away from processed foods, sugar and grains and eat fresh, whole foods including lean meats or beans/lentils, nuts, vegetables, fruits, oils, some dairy and plenty of water. If you do this, I believe you will be completely amazed at how much better you feel and how much better your body functions!

Warehouse Clubs

A great way to save money on nutrient-dense, healthy food is to become a member of a warehouse club like Costco or Sam's Club. Buying fruits, vegetables and lean meats in bulk is essentially an unsurpassed method to save tons of cash! Usually these foods are all located on the back wall along the perimeter of the store so they can be easily restocked.

Warehouse clubs are one of the main sources of fresh, bulk ingredients and whole foods that supply local restaurants so you can use this to your advantage and stock up on ingredients for you and your family. These stores also have healthy bulk ingredients like olive oil, avocado oil and other items such as beans and fresh eggs.

Many people say, "yeah, but a membership costs money!" Yep, but the small annual fee is ridiculously low compared to the money you'll save during an entire year! A great trick is to get a membership and then add relatives or friends onto your membership. Simply split the annual membership fee amongst all the cardholders and the price drops drastically! For warehouse clubs, make a list of the main foods you use, buy them in bulk and then split the food and cost. This way, you're getting these foods at the best price and you aren't wasting food by having some of it spoil before it gets used. Some, if not most, of your friends and neighbors have the same challenge of using larger amounts of food when they buy in bulk. Plan ahead and everyone can benefit by splitting up large packages of various items.

"Don't dig your grave with your own knife and fork."
~English Proverb

A word of warning, avoid going to these stores when they have "sample days." The samples are never slices of a fresh apple or a handful of green snap peas; they are always heavily processed foods which usually cost much more than their whole food counterparts. There is a reason they need to give out free samples, if you ever really looked at the ingredient list you'd never buy them. They give you samples so you taste it first and then have your brain override your common sense and end up buying it. Be smart.

Local Farmers and Ranchers

Now, more than ever, we are realizing the critical importance of local farmers and ranchers who are able to bring freshly harvested fruits, vegetables and meats to our local markets or farmer's markets. These health-conscious families understand the critical role our food contributes to our health as a community and society. As our society has unfortunately changed to a more convenience and processed food lifestyle, we have almost lost touch with our local farmers and ranchers who have faithfully served our communities for generations. They were the original source of fresh produce and meats and still serve their neighbors and communities to this day. I encourage you to make an effort to go visit your local farmers and ranchers who have stands either at their property or at the local farmer's market. It's an awesome experience and helping your neighbors helps you as well.

Many farmers and ranchers will often sell their organic, grass-fed livestock directly to customers. You can buy a third, half or full beef or pork directly from the rancher and have it delivered after it has been butchered and wrapped. All it takes is a small, efficient freezer and you'll have organic meat for a year! Their offerings are very reasonably priced and generally less expensive than most grocery chains. By supporting farmers and ranchers you are supporting your community and neighbors. Most importantly, you'll know exactly where your meat came from and can rest easy knowing it wasn't processed, mixed with fillers or dyed for color.

If you live in a medium to large city and this concept seems strange to you, feel free to go visit some of the farmers markets in the rural areas where some of the vendors can point you in the right direction. Purchasing meat this way has been in existence as long as humans have been forming communities and co-ops. I truly enjoy visiting with local farmers and ranchers to see which crops are in season or livestock might be available for me to buy in order to provide my family with nutrient-dense food. By supporting our local farmers and ranchers we are insuring a healthy future for our future generations.

Another great source of whole, fresh food can be grown in your own local garden. More and more urban garden areas are being formed each year in cities and neighborhoods. Growing your own garden vegetables and fruit is a neat way to learn more about the food you eat. Gardening is incredibly rewarding especially if you have children who can learn important lessons and have a sense of responsibility for their garden, too. It takes some planning and organization but the results taste great! Simply go online and search for phrases such as "starting a garden" or "how to start a garden" and you'll be able to get started right now!

Ultimately, by maximizing the combination of perimeter shopping, buying from local farmers and ranchers, or maybe having your own garden, you'll be eating foods in their original, unaltered states which will automatically allow you to eat much healthier and save money.

Organic or Not-Organic, That is The Question

Another very common question I get concerning how to eat healthier and not spend as much shopping is whether or not to buy only organic foods. The goal is to reduce the amount of dangerous and unhealthy chemicals you are consuming. This is always a controversial conversation but I think it comes down to a couple main issues. The first point I like to make is if you are currently consuming lots of processed, prepackaged foods than you are consuming TONS of chemicals, preservatives, additives and dyes as ingredients in the processed foods. In addition, you are consuming all kinds of pesticides, herbicides and fungicides used on the various ingredients while they were growing before they ever even made it into the processed food. Many of the ingredients in processed foods were either produced in a chemical facility or grown in fields without organic methods so you're already getting exposed to a significant amount of the bad stuff when eating processed foods.

As you are modifying your shopping and eating habits as part of your nutritional plan, you need to realize that by changing to more whole, naturally grown food, you are already likely getting a significant reduction in the number of dangerous chemicals you are consuming, even if you don't buy organically grown foods. So, the choice whether to eat only organic really comes down to the issue of cost. Organic food is expensive and often times spoils more quickly due to the lack of preservatives present in and on the food.

I recommend not buying organic foods as you change your nutrition plan as the high cost creates a negative mental feeling when grocery shopping. I recommend avoiding all organic and buying regular whole, natural foods initially. Once you've made these changes to your nutrition plan, then you can decide if you want to change over to all organic versions of these foods. After a decent length of time eating healthier and increasing your activity, you'll likely have a surplus of extra cash you've saved by not wasting it on restaurants, medications, health care bills since you're now healthier! Use this extra cash on buying organic if you want! Cha-ching!

Healthy Tip: Make sure you wash your vegetables and fruits to get off as many sprayed on chemicals as possible. This old saying easily explains this principle: the solution to pollution is dilution. Aggressively rinsing and sometimes brushing the outside of fresh foods will remove chemicals and dirt from the harvest process.

Counting Calories

Whether or not you choose to count calories is up to you. Most people find it labor intensive and time consuming. Most people don't make the time to balance their bank accounts so how many people are going to keep track of every calorie, every day? Not many. I personally don't recommend counting calories because I don't think it provides very much value for most people unless you have an analytical mind and like number crunching. The reason I don't generally recommend that people count calories is because it is not really the calories which seem to matter as much as the quality of the calories.

For example, 200 calories of a candy bar versus 200 calories of a green pepper are metabolized very differently and affect the health of your body very differently. When the pure sugar of candy enters your system, it causes an enormous spike in both your blood sugar and the fat storage hormone insulin. The spike in insulin causes your body to try and store those calories as fat, which is NOT what you want. And, your hunger center will be stimulated and you'll feel hungry again within minutes to an hour. This is why most people graze or eat up to six meals during the day. By eating so many carbs, you're telling your body its starving and to store fat all at the same time. This makes us eat more since we're constantly hungry.

Compare this to the 200 calories of green pepper which does not cause a large spike in blood sugar and insulin and therefore doesn't prompt your body to try and store it as fat. This reduces weight gain, which IS what you want. Also, the vegetable has a lot of fiber which is great for your digestive system. And, if you measure out 200 calories of green pepper, you'll realize it is A LOT of green pepper and goes a long way compared to the speck of candy for the same amount of calories.

If you are going to eat 200 calories, wouldn't you rather eat the version which allows you to eat more, feel better, digest better, and not promote putting more fat on your body?

I really don't care about the number of calories you consume; what I care about is the where you get the calories from.

Don't get me wrong, I understand the calories in/calories out theory as well as the benefits of calculating your Basal Metabolic Rate. But in the big picture, it takes a lot of time to add up calories each and every day. Sure, many people say that focusing on the calories you consume helps you examine and realize which foods you are eating. There is no doubt this can be helpful but whether someone actually does it or not is the deciding factor.

Also, this is another common form of adding an additional habit to another habit, or habit stacking, which can end up sabotaging your good intentions. In other words, if you require yourself to track every calorie every time you eat then you will end up spending a lot of unnecessary time focusing on food which can create a bad cycle. If you buy healthy foods and only have these available, you won't have to worry about what you're eating since you already know and have planned ahead to set yourself up for success! If you see the forest for the trees you'll have a lot better chance at reaching your goals.

Daily Multivitamin

One of the best habits to have regarding your daily nutrition is to take a high quality, daily multivitamin. This is the least costly habit which yields some of the highest nutritional benefit available. Don't waste your money on the gummy ones as it is another example of companies adding sugar and chemicals to a normally healthy product.

The best time to your take multivitamin is in the evening or before bed. Think about it, if you are eating well during the day then your body is absorbing all of the vitamins and minerals from the healthy food you are eating so you won't be able to absorb much more. Since you aren't eating and are fasting while you sleep, taking your multivitamin at night will increase the chance it gets absorbed and can contribute to your overall health. Again, try to find a higher quality daily multivitamin as there are many low quality ones with lots of useless fillers and various forms of the vitamins which have low ability to be absorbed by your body. Ask a pharmacist about which brands or types they recommend. Pharmacists are literally experts in medications and are able to offer their expertise to the general public on pretty much any medication or vitamin question. We often see pharmacists busy behind the counter or glass working on certain prescriptions however every pharmacist I know genuinely enjoys educating and helping people in their effort to become healthier.

Powders, Pills and Promises

Supplements have become a ridiculously enormous industry in the United States alone. It's difficult to tell exactly how much since there are weak regulations on what is considered a supplement but Americans likely spend around $30-35 BILLION of their hard-earned dollars per year. This is completely ridiculous! Various supplements such as protein powders, herbal supplements and weightlifting products offer to replace or add something that is missing and "supplement" your nutrition plan so you can function at a higher level. I have patients who can barely afford their utility bills but always tell me which new protein supplement they bought. I always have to ask, "Do you even know if you are low on protein?" They never know how to answer because it never occurs to many people that they likely don't need to supplement a single nutrient.

Please think about it like this: if you are eating a healthy mix of whole, fresh foods including meats, vegetables, fruit, some dairy and a quality multivitamin then you are likely getting all the nutrients including protein, minerals, and vitamins you will ever need. Supplements aren't necessary unless you are eating poor quality, processed food which has had all of the nutrients removed!

The food and supplement industries have created a clever and high profit business model: remove nutrients from healthy, whole food which results in expensive, processed food and then sell a version of these nutrients back to you in the form of an expensive, questionable supplement! It's brilliant and unfortunately, we're buying it! Also, the supplement industry is so poorly monitored these products can contain ingredients which could be dangerous to adults, children and pregnant women. I see patients every year who are unknowingly consuming toxic levels of vitamin D and various herbal supplements believing they are doing the right thing.

Protein supplements have become very popular over the past decade as well. High protein intake over a short period of time can be really tough on your kidneys. Taking protein supplements above and beyond a healthy consumption of lean meat is likely adding too much protein to your nutrition plan. If you are wondering if you even need more protein you can always ask your primary care provider who can order a simple blood test.

In conclusion, I'm simply asking you to be wise and really think about why you are taking a supplement and if you even truly need it. One of my favorite human metabolism professors used to joke that supplements are simply expensive urine. If you're eating healthy and you already absorb all the nutrients you need, then any additional nutrients or supplements are simply sent out with the waste and end up being just that, a waste.

Increase Fiber

An easy way to decrease the amount of low quality processed foods while increasing your intake of healthy foods is to increase your daily fiber intake. Whole foods such as vegetables and fruits naturally contain a high amount of fiber when eaten with their skins still attached and in their whole form. Strive to increase your consumption of foods such as apples, carrots, broccoli, cauliflower, and green salads. Fiber is also known to help decrease the risk of some types of cancers.

If you find yourself grazing or snacking throughout the day, then you will definitely benefit from packing fiber-filled foods to snack on. Simply slice up a couple apples, a handful of snap peas, or make some carrot sticks and you'll feel full throughout the day and won't even be interested in the office snack machine or candy jar. Simple tricks like packing some sliced fruit and vegetables can be a game changer if you find yourself pulled away from your work duties due to hunger throughout the day. Most workplaces have employee lunchrooms with refrigerators to store your lunch. My trick is to slice up a bunch of raw carrot sticks, green peppers, and celery sticks in a reusable, gallon size Ziploc. I also put some apple and cucumber slices in another Ziploc and take it to the office at the beginning of the week. This way, I don't have to pack this each night for the next day which saves a lot of time. As long as you seal it between uses it will easily last all week. I generally rinse and reuse the plastic bags, which saves money and also saves space in the landfill for your sugar-filled processed foods you just removed from your cupboards...hint, hint. Also, a bunch of bananas, walnuts, pecans, peanuts and dried fruit easily pack and store at the office for snacks. Trail mix is a great option, too. Using these tricks you'll save time, money and be more productive whether you work for a boss or yourself as your own boss!

Another huge benefit of consuming fruit and vegetables is their water content. These foods will help you stay hydrated by providing natural water intake. Some people really have a tough time staying hydrated so this is a great method to use if this applies to you. If you fill your stomach with nutritious foods you won't feel the need to fill it with junk food.

Back in the day we used to eat a salad before having the main course and coincidentally we didn't have the same rates of obesity and diabetes as we do now. Consider restarting this tradition since it's a healthy way to feel full more quickly and reduce the amount of the calorie-dense, main course you'll eat. You can easily buy spinach, lettuce, peppers, and olives in bulk at your local warehouse store. These ingredients will create a great salad to have before or part of your lunch and dinner. It's easy to eat your greens when you're hungry before main meals. Make it a habit and it'll feel really strange not having a fresh salad before your main course!

Learn How to Cook For Free

The lack of cooking knowledge has prevented younger generations from inexpensively eating well. Purchasing bulk foods and cooking at home is probably the number one way to save money and be healthier. These days I recommend going online to find fun, free videos to learn how to cook better. (Of course there are a lot of cooking shows on cable TV these days but who would waste their money or time watching cable TV in the first place.)

There are hundreds of cookbooks available in print and online to learn recipes and methods for low carb or no carb cooking. Learn easily from the professionals and you'll be cooking healthier in no time! Consider visiting your local library for a FREE library card and access to thousands of FREE cookbooks and food magazines!

YouTube has tons of free cooking videos which help you learn pretty much any technique or method of cooking you could ever imagine. Cook along with the videos and improve your skills without spending a dime on books or lessons! Getting healthy and losing weight doesn't have to cost you anything, in fact, you'll save money!

You can make learning to cook a fun social event with friends or family as well. If you're learning together, simply divide the grocery list up and have each person bring certain ingredients for a great dish! Gather at someone's home and either make the dish together or if one of you knows how to do it, have them demonstrate and teach you how to make it! This fun evening is inexpensive, social, and gives you a new skill!

Another great way to learn how to cook is to have a group of friends who go from home to home in an evening with each location responsible for making a different course of the meal! This is really a blast if you all live within biking distance of one another. At the first home, the host may show everyone how they have learned to make a specific, fresh salad. At the second home you might learn how to cook the main course. At another home you can learn how to make a low carb, low sugar dessert to end the night! It's a great way to spend an evening with friends and also helps build friendships while learning new skills together!

Get a Drink of Water

Drinking a full glass of water 5-10 minutes before each meal is a great way to feel full earlier and also stay hydrated. Your stomach has pressure sensors which tell you when you're full. By starting out your meal with a glass of water, this provides a zero calorie head start and when you do eat, you'll feel full earlier and won't be able to eat as much as you might otherwise. Plus, you get the added benefit of staying hydrated which allows your body to function at an optimal level. The salad plates made by most every dinnerware manufacturer are the ideal size plate for most people. I recommend avoiding the large size plates found in dinnerware sets. They are simply too large to eat meals on consistently and will absolutely cause you to overeat.

Smaller Plate

Many weight loss experts recommend using a smaller plate at meals. This has proven to be an easy way to monitor the amount of food you eat and provides a psychological advantage to you. Your brain feels like it is eating a lot when your meal fills your plate. So, if the plate is smaller you are consuming less food. Eating lean meats combined with fresh vegetables can quickly fill up a plate.

An awesome tip for packing your lunch is to have a specific size lunch container which won't allow you to pack too much extra food into it. I'm a big fan of some of the Bento boxes available online. Using one of these you'll be able to set your portion sizes very easily. I bought a set of five lunch containers with lids online for about $10 and have used them every day for over two years! Don't set yourself up for failure by packing too much food and feeling tempted to eat it all.

Share a Meal with Someone

If you do end up visiting a restaurant, consider ordering a regular meal but splitting it in half so you get the pleasure of dining out with less cost and less food intake. Most importantly, you get the luxury of spending some quality time with a friend or family member! Awhile back there was a book written about this principle and the benefits of making your lunch time productive to nurture relationships while enjoying some healthy food. The old adage of "breaking bread" with someone really does help a relationship grow. Many restaurants will allow anyone to order off the "seniors" menu which is great since these are always smaller portions, too.

Food Dependence

"If hunger is not the problem,
then eating is not the solution."
~Unknown

Many people eat for comfort and to avoid being social. Consider speaking to your primary care provider if there are mental, emotional, and social issues you feel you are trying to solve by eating. This is VERY common and is often overlooked in our society. Many people eat when they are bored as well which can be a big source of extra eating and ultimately weight gain. Many patients I work with have realized they were only eating most of their extra meals and snacks to soothe emotional and traumatic psychological wounds instead of dealing with them. If you feel like you are an emotional eater which is limiting your ability to reach your goals, consider finding a counselor through your work, church or community center. A skilled counselor is incredibly helpful to assist you in evaluating your psychological dependence on food and can help improve your relationship with food and help reach your goals. Never feel embarrassed or too proud to seek assistance from someone more knowledgeable when it comes to your mental and physical health. The act of bravery is to be supported and commended and should never be a negative feeling. Again, this is much more common than people think so know you are not alone if this applies to you.

CHAPTER 5

AVOID THESE HABITS!

Face it, our lifestyles are generally filled with habits which likely aren't supporting our goals! I recommend you really take an honest look at your current habits and decide whether they are ultimately worth keeping, modifying, or getting rid of all together. When reviewing these habits, really think about where they are ultimately leading to and if you actually get any benefit out of them. It's amazing how many people I see self-sabotage their health and self-neglect their bodies in the name of convenience and habit.

Convenience Store Habit

These days we live in the Golden Age of Convenience. Everything is designed to be fast and convenient so we can get on with our busy, yet unproductive, lives. Convenience stores are a major source of sabotage for your healthy lifestyle plan.

They are everywhere; on every corner, in every neighborhood, in every community in the nation! The shelves are stocked with the most comprehensive collection of unhealthy, processed "food products" I've been describing including candy bars, soda pop, energy drinks, sugary coffees, beer and chips. These stores have the highest density of carbohydrate-based foods on the planet! These foods are highly processed and have no nutrition whatsoever. They are poor quality, highly marketed products designed to be able to sit on the shelf for months and years without spoiling. Convenience stores are essentially the smaller, more condensed version of the larger grocery store aisles.

If you want the easiest way to remember how to eat less processed foods, less carbohydrates and to get healthier, remember this rule: if the food you are considering eating is usually found in a convenience store, don't eat it. That's it. That's all you need to know. You'll thank me later.

The other reason I urge people to not use convenience stores is the financial cost. Since the convenience products are designed for easy transport and individual servings, they require a greater amount of expensive packaging which increases the cost to you, the consumer. These stores are designed to sell single servings of products which are sometimes 50-200% more expensive than buying bulk food. Save your cash and take a pass!

The only way you'll ever lose any weight going to convenience stores is by emptying out your hard-earned cash from your wallet!

Sports drinks are another source of pure, unhealthy sugar with a couple healthy sounding vitamins added in so they are disguised as a health food. They are completely overpriced sugar water and if you are eating healthy foods, they have zero benefit and the sugar in these products is likely making you sick. Energy drinks are another source of extra sugar and chemicals our younger generations seem to seek out. I recommend avoiding these as much as possible to reduce exposure to sugar, artificial sweeteners and chemicals. Premade, bottled coffee drinks like mocha and vanilla flavors from major coffee makers are also complete garbage as they provide essentially no nutritional benefits, contain a bunch of empty sugar and calories, and actually don't have much caffeine compared to plain, cheap drip coffee. Avoid them at all costs.

I realize sometimes there is no choice but to stop at a convenience store, especially if you are traveling. I urge you to search high and low for a fruit basket which is usually hidden between the candy rack and the donuts. Grab a banana or an apple instead of a king-size candy bar and cola drink. Also, if you need to put fuel in your car then simply pay at the pump, don't go into the store, and drive away in your car as fast as you can!

One of the most disappointing things I see on my commute in the morning is essentially the same set of cars and trucks parked outside the convenience stores. I know these folks have stopped to find something to eat on the way to work. How can a person expect to feel well and be able to get work completed when their breakfast is a bag of powdered donuts and large soda? It baffles my mind. Not to mention the fact they are paying a "convenience tax" for expensive, convenience foods they likely can't honestly afford. I believe if they really thought about it, they would choose not to pay the extra cost. I truly believe if they took only one hour per week and grocery shopped ahead of time at a warehouse store, they would save tons of money! And, no doubt their work would improve because they are fueling their bodies with nutrients and quality food. And since they wouldn't have to stop for something to eat every day, they would either be able to spend more time with their family before work since they don't have to leave as early. Or, they could leave at the same time and get to work early or at least on time, which is never a bad thing!

Unhealthy Snacking Habit

"The bigger snacks mean bigger slacks."
~Unknown

Snacking is an all-too-easy source of extra calories throughout the day. There are so many convenience foods available today it boggles my mind. Food products including candy, chips, and soda are easy sources of unhealthy calories, carbohydrates and chemicals. Snacking on junk food sabotages you two main ways; the first is because you are eating highly processed, carbohydrate-based foods which we know are harming your health. Secondly, these foods are quickly broken down by your stomach which causes a spike in insulin. This makes you hungry again which causes the cycle to repeat itself, all day long, year after year and decade after decade. This situation is the last thing you need if you are trying to lose weight, get healthier or improve your blood sugars.

"What you eat in private
will show up in public."
~Unknown

The easiest and most healthy solution to unhealthy snacking is to provide your own snacks so you don't have to go on a "carb search" throughout your day. Once most people have the first taste of something sweet or high carbohydrate, their brain goes on a search for more and the cycle perpetuates. Think about it, you're fine all day if you don't take something from the candy dish. But, as soon as you do, its game over and you'll go back until it's either empty or someone starts harassing you about it. Right? Right.

I mentioned this before but it's worth repeating; when you are at the warehouse store, be sure to buy some big bags of vegetables such as snap peas, carrots, celery, a bag of apples, oranges, or bananas. Also, get some bulk almonds, pistachios, trail mix or peanuts to add into your snacks for variety. This simple habit gives you the control of eating and enjoying the foods you know are healthy and contributing nutrients to your body and you won't have to wonder if the stale, last remaining, two-day-old donut on the table is worth the risk to your health. Humans are too advanced to have to make such stressful survival decisions like this in a day. Besides, it also saves you tons of cash. It's ridiculously inexpensive to eat healthy snacks if you buy in bulk and do very minimal preparation for the week. An added benefit is you won't have to leave your work area as often which allows you to be more effective and get more done. Why support your local candy and junk food vendor if you could be supporting your own bank account!

Daily Coffee Habit

A costly habit affecting millions of us during the work week is stopping for a morning coffee at a drive thru stand or a major chain location. Many people purchase blended coffees and baked goods on their way to work. Blended coffees are chemical bombs. You might as well have a morning milkshake and stop pretending it's a coffee. Check out the major chains' websites and look at all of the sugar and fillers they add to these "coffees." A large blended coffee at one major chain has over 1000 calories and over 50 grams of sugar! If I have to tell you this is completely stupid then forget it, you've already lost. It is your personal responsibility to take care of your body and avoid consuming these unhealthy food products which are slowly killing you. Let's all stop pretending these socially acceptable "food products" are worth consuming.

Your coffee habit also has a high financial cost. A popular personal finance writer described this obvious waste of money over about five books that you can look up while you're in the drive-thru getting your 1000 calorie "coffee." Essentially, if you spend an average of $5 per day for a basic working year you'll end up spending about $1000 per year on just this one bad habit. Over ten years that's $10,000. That's a decent chunk of change you could be spending on yourself or your family. Can you imagine having this amount in your bank account accruing interest instead of spending it on junk food? Use your money for good instead of evil and think about the money you spend on food as buying nutrients and you'll likely be more careful with your spending. When it comes to high priced coffees, a lot of my patients say, "but that's my treat!" How is eating sugar-filled, junk food you just bought in a 6,000 pound SUV after idling in a drive thru for ten minutes a treat in any possible way? Here's a treat: get healthier, ride your bike, save some cash and take better care of yourself and your family. Now THAT'S a treat.

Restaurant Habit

On average, it is estimated Americans spend $3,000 per year on eating outside their home! In 2016, the CDC notes that food and drink sales in America totaled over $766,000,000,000. Yep, that's BILLIONS!

The average American eats out 5-7 times per week, which is crazy. That's eating out at least once almost every day! Besides the obvious financial cost, this habit is costing us our health and futures. It's clear that most Americans, especially younger generations, don't like to cook or frankly don't know how. Restaurants don't care about your health or waistline, they care about their bottom line. I recommend you really try to avoid eating outside of your own kitchen as often and you'll quickly see the various benefits including your smaller waist line and your larger bank account balance. Besides, who really knows how much hair, bugs, spit and who knows what is actually in and on the food you eat at restaurants and fast food joints. I don't know and frankly I don't want to know. It's good to know what is in, and not in, your food and making meals at home guarantees this.

If you do go out to restaurants, the trick is to really evaluate the foods on the menu. Often, there is a "healthy choice" section of the menu. Unfortunately, even the "healthy" choices like salads often have more calories than a plain old cheeseburger. If you do get a burger consider ordering it without the bun and use lettuce as a wrap instead. Some fast food chains have created healthy menus with fruits and veggies. This is great, although you are probably paying 3-4 times more for the same ingredients you could buy at the grocery store or farmer's market.

Another issue with restaurant meals is the portion size. In order to satisfy hungry, carb-craving patrons, restaurants work hard to keep their portions large, which is great unless you're trying to lose weight or get healthier. The best trick here is to eat a third to a half of your meal and ask for a to-go box. That way you can enjoy your meal with your family or friends and also have left-overs for the next day's lunch or dinner. Also, ask your server if there are "half" portions or a senior's version of the meal you were interested in ordering. Many times, these are smaller portions and less expensive. It's a win-win situation.

Fast Food Habit

Most researchers and experts attribute our obesity epidemic to eating significantly higher amounts of fast food over the past several decades. Fast food chains have become a primary source of meals for many Americans and tend to be frequented by the people lowest on the socioeconomic scale, in other words, poor people. It's essentially a huge tax on the poor. These high carb, calorie-rich foods are the absolute worse kinds of prepared food you can buy. Fast food chains are experts at delivering fast, unhealthy food at low prices in an efficient manner. Their "food" is made of the lowest quality ingredients and has been processed so much there is generally very little nutritional value. Also, many "meals" can cost up to $10 PER PERSON, PER MEAL! How is this less expensive than bulk, whole food? As a population we have become overfed, but undernourished, due to the high calorie and high carbohydrate fast food dependent lifestyle.

The other downfall of fast food is it takes essentially no effort to obtain meals containing thousands of calories, fat, salt and sugar. You don't even have to get out of your car to get a meal. We can even order pizzas, sandwiches and burgers over the internet and have it delivered right to our door! The best rule for this is: under no circumstances should you ever buy food that comes through a window!

Alcohol Habit

Alcohol is a depressant and in the big picture it really doesn't have any positive benefit to a person's health. The use of alcohol is one of the most common forms of self-neglect and self-sabotage I see in people since it is so socially acceptable and a big part of people's social lives. Sure, it's nice to go out for a drink with friends every once in a while but ultimately your health and weight loss progress will be significantly reduced with the use/abuse of alcohol. Alcohol has the potential to add lots extra calories to your daily caloric intake, often 100-300 calories PER DRINK! So, if the average person has 2-3 drinks while out on the town or at home, this can add an easy 300-900 calories to your daily intake, just in alcohol! Sure, maybe you plan to go for one drink and then leave. Usually what happens is that you end up having one... after another! In my opinion, the use of alcohol isn't really a calorie issue but more of a big picture issue. Alcohol increases your risk of some cancers, bad decisions, and is a costly habit financially as well. Avoid the situation and save your health and cash while increasing your productivity for the next day!

By the way, drinking alcohol really dehydrates you and is one side effect of alcohol which doesn't get as much attention as it deserves. You may notice your urine is dark yellow after having some alcohol due to the dehydrating effects of alcohol. Your body needs to be hydrated to optimally function. The next day after consuming alcohol you're often dehydrated, bloated, and probably hungover. At this point, it' helpful to realize alcohol is preventing you from reaching your goals. Consider helping yourself by taking a break from alcohol for several months. During this time, keep track of your weight because all other things being equal, you're likely to have much easier weight loss and overall feel much better!

Smoking Habit

If you smoke cigarettes, my goal isn't to make you feel bad about smoking as I'm sure everyone around you already does. My goal for discussing smoking is to help you realize one important perspective explaining why you likely still smoke cigarettes. Working with patients who smoke over the years has taught me one thing – the reason they smoke actually isn't completely due to the nicotine or even the oral fixation of smoking.

The reason smokers smoke is because smoking is the one thing throughout their entire life which they have been able to rely on and has never failed them or let them down. Maybe spouses have come and gone, jobs were fine and then they weren't and happiness came and went but the one solid, support they have always been able to rely on has been their cigarettes. Think about it, when a smoker goes for a cigarette, they're often stressed or nervous about something, or perhaps they simply need a break from the current situation for time to think and chill out. If a smoker is almost anywhere in our society, it has been socially acceptable for them to leave a situation and go smoke. THIS is the underlying psychological reason many people still smoke cigarettes.

If you smoke, I'm asking you to really think about this. One of the best ways for someone to quit smoking is to ask them to pay attention to the moment when they think about needing to go for a cigarette. What is happening in that moment that triggers you to need to leave and go out for a cigarette? Once you realize what your triggers are, it becomes very easy to avoid these triggers. Also, replace smoking a cigarette with a walk down to the corner and back, calling a friend for a minute or even checking social media. All of these are healthier habit replacements for the unhealthy habit of smoking. Give it a try and you just might find this is the answer you've been looking for to finally stop smoking.

Finishing Your Plate Habit

This habit has been ingrained in most Americans since we were children. How many times did you hear your parents say, "Finish your plate, because there are people starving in other countries." I heard it almost daily as a kid. As a result, I still have difficulty leaving food on my plate, even though I'm full. It is a habit which can be a disastrous to someone trying to lose weight or become healthier. The solution: leave food on your plate, it is absolutely okay! That's right, I said to leave food on your plate and don't feel guilty. Or, better yet, dish up smaller portions during your meals so you don't have to leave food on your plate in the first place. Or, pack the leftovers for lunch tomorrow! Being polite and finishing everything on your plate has the possibility of adding several pounds to your weight per week. Over a couple months, you could be 5-10 pounds lighter with just this one simple habit change!

Eating Fast Habit

How many of us have gulped down breakfast on the way to work or sat in a parking lot near our office to eat the fast food lunch? The problem with eating fast is because our stomachs have pressure receptors that signal when we are full. It is very easy to trick these receptors if we eat fast and generally results in overeating. Most studies show if someone eats slower, these receptors are more accurate at gauging how full the stomach is and signaling it's time to stop eating. Slow down while you eat, enjoy your food, savor the taste and don't be in a rush. You'll feel better and your waistline with thank you.

Nutrition Summary

I recommend you take a few minutes and add up the financial cost of all the processed food products, various supplements and protein powders, restaurant receipts and convenience store purchases so you can truly realize how much money you are spending on the effort to provide yourself nutrients each month. This monthly price tag is very high for most people and unfortunately, all we are buying ourselves is illness and bigger waistlines as there is also a significant health cost to you as well. Instead of working so hard and spending so much to buy low quality processed foods in an effort to provide nutrients, I encourage you to simply buy fresh, whole food which will provide everything your body needs to be healthy and function at the highest level and you won't have to use expensive, questionable supplements!

I realize by discussing nutrition and which foods to eat and which to avoid, I am essentially wandering into one of the most heated topics for debate and discussion that exists rivalled only by politics, religion and relationships! I do this willingly and knowingly because I think it's the right thing to do. When I recommend significantly decreasing or limiting certain foods like carbohydrates, especially whole grains and processed foods, people always seem to lose their minds and immediately ask about ten questions to try and play "gotcha" with me. What about athletes or runners or people who need carbs due to a disease, they ask. My answer is always the same: when discussing these principles I'm talking about the 99.99% of unhealthy, overweight Americans who are not athletes, runners, or those with a specific metabolic disease. I speak in absolutes such as "always" and "never" because the individuals who require daily carbohydrates already know who they are and only comprise a very small percentage of the population. Our bodies can convert proteins and fats into carbohydrates or create carbohydrates if needed which is why we truly do not need to consume daily carbohydrates, though the "experts" still indicate at least half of our daily food is carbohydrate. As I like to say, what could possibly go wrong?

Let's stop talking about the exceptions and start talking about the vast majority of us who need to reevaluate our priorities and focus in order to improve our health and quality of life. Everyone is exceptional, but most people are rarely the exceptions.

CHAPTER 6

GET ACTIVE!

"Those who think they have not time for bodily exercise will sooner or later have to find time for illness."
~Edward Stanley

I challenge you to change your perspective about exercise. For most people, saying the word "exercise" gives us the same queasy stomach feeling as "IRS, taxes, or lawyer." Instead of instantly imagining barbells, fitness clubs, and expensive personal trainers, consider another option. Consider being physically active, not necessarily exercising. When people decide they want to get healthier and lose some weight, they start by researching the newest and usually expensive workout programs, local fitness facilities, and they also look online for expensive exercise equipment. Again, in order to make progress or show commitment most people feel like they need to lay some serious cash down to start the process. This is completely wrong. In fact, it is literally working against your success and results. I'm not saying personal trainers, gym memberships or buying workout programs and equipment won't help at all or can't be effective. What I'm saying is it is often unnecessary and expensive. After you've been active or working out for a month or two, you may feel ready to get more intense and focused on your activities or workouts. At that point, it makes complete sense to consider hiring someone to help or buying a program or product to move you forward with the habits you've already formed. My perspective is to start simple and low cost and only then should you proceed with getting more complicated and expensive. Find an activity such as a daily walk, bike ride or a light weight program you can do at home for free. Do this DAILY for a month or two to get your body used to the activity. This will help your endurance, flexibility, and strength while preventing injury. Also, the activity doesn't have to the same every day. Maybe one day you walk to the store and the next you ride your bike to a friend's house.

> *"A man's health can be judged by*
> *which he takes two at a time – pills or stairs."*
> ~Joan Welsh

Our bodies are remarkable machines which require daily physical activity to maintain overall function and longevity. Many diseases which plague us today were much less prevalent even 50-100 years ago. Conditions such as Type 2 diabetes and obesity were significantly less prevalent in the past. The combination of high calorie foods combined with a sedentary lifestyle is the 1-2 punch to our health and waistlines.

Our bodies work best when we are able to be physically active each and every day. For example, blood flow to limbs has been found to improve with activity. Our joints, muscles, tendons and ligaments hydrate and function properly when we're are active. Our bones stay dense and strong which reduces the chance of breaking by working against gravity and moving. This is demonstrated by astronauts who live for any length of time in space. Their bones will become less dense due to lack of resistance in a weightless environment. Our lungs function by using a combination of muscles and more importantly pressure changes. When you are physically moving your chest and lungs are able to expand and move air more easily. The lack of physical activity is the reason for the fast decline of someone's health when they are bed-ridden.

My medical colleagues and I often use sayings including, "motion is lotion" and "if you rest, you rust." These accurately describe the mindset you should have when thinking about ways to incorporate more activity into your life. If people only stopped to consider all of the enormous benefits being physically active daily provide a person, they'd never sit still. Again, looking at the big picture of why you want to get healthy makes your decisions pretty easy. Even though you may want to become more active to lose weight or reverse a medical condition, the benefits of physical activity are universally beneficial to every organ and system in your body.

Being physically active is a remarkable thing. There are no other therapies, drugs, or technology which can provide the enormous benefits to our health, waistline and future as being physically active. You should make it a simple habit to be active for at least 15-30 minutes daily by incorporating movement into an activity you already do every day.

By making it every day you are removing the decision component and it becomes automatic. We all know if something is to be completed 5 days per week, it eventually turns into 3 days per week and within no time becomes, "wait, what am I supposed to be doing again?"

The current guidelines indicate all Americans, even those with disabilities, those who are pregnant, the elderly and children should be getting between 150-300 minutes per week of activity. ANY ACTIVITY, EVERY DAY. Preferably moderate intensity activity but ANY will do. The previous guidelines published a decade ago recommended activity in about 10 minute intervals. That minimum has actually been removed since most Americans are getting so little activity and movement in their day that experts can't even set a minimum block of time any longer! Currently, about 80% of Americans are not active enough and it is only going to get worse.

Being sedentary or sitting is the worst thing you can do during the day. Most of our days are spent sitting while at work, while driving/commuting, eating, watching TV, playing video games, and using a computer; and it is slowly killing us. Between the years 1940-1960, our lives quickly started to become more sedentary. Cars became much more affordable and easy for an American family to own. Also, television started showing up in most homes and families started tuning in to programs and the evening news. Housewives started watching soap operas in the afternoons which were literally dramas with commercials selling soap!

"Movement is a medicine for creating change
in a person's physical, emotional, and mental states."
~Carol Welch

For most people, the risk of not being physically active is far more dangerous than the risk of starting to become active after being sedentary. That said, if you have a history of heart attack, stroke or chronic conditions, I recommend seeing your health care provider for a quick check and to help set up an activity plan. I really can't think of anyone who would be at high risk while going for a walk down the block and back to begin being active, but be smart, and if there is any question in your mind about being evaluated prior to getting more active, then get evaluated.

Being required to put in a disclaimer like this is irritating to me since there is going to be a group of you who read this and think, "Oh, I can't start getting active until I check with my health care provider and since I can't get in for several months, I guess it will have to wait." This gives you a way out and allows you to postpone getting active. If this applies to you, stand up and go walk down the block and back. Again, everyone is exceptional, but most people are rarely the exceptions. No health care provider in their right mind is going to argue against this as long as you use common sense and you have someone around or helping you. I've never seen the cause of death on a death certificate say "Walked around block." Every day you postpone getting moving is another day you get further behind. Everyone's situation is different so just use common sense and get going already. Find some basic life activity you generally need to do most days of the week, like going to the mailbox, and start walking instead of driving to get it done. You'll be shocked at how much benefit this gives you physically, mentally, and emotionally.

Technology can be a huge advantage when we are working to become healthier and lose weight. Your ability to search online and instantly find exercise programs, yoga programs, nutrition information and general information to become healthier is unparalleled. There are now activity trackers, smart watches, and apps you can use to help reach your goals. While you may find these helpful, I don't recommend buying any of them, yet. There are great free apps you can use to track your activities and these will be sufficient for 99% of people getting started. Only after you can go 5 miles or be active for at least an hour should you buy any sort of widget to use. Again, by buying the must-have new watch, activity band or software, you are shifting the responsibility and initiative of being active onto the technology or device instead of yourself. I recommend avoiding this temptation and only buying the gadget once you have already established the daily habit. Maybe buy this device or app as a reward for being active 30 days in a row! Who said this had to be boring and no fun?

As I mentioned, the benefits of being physically active on a daily basis are vast and improve essentially every aspect of your health by optimizing the function of your body systems and organs. Below is just a small list of the benefits I am referring to. Prepare to have your mind blown!

Here are the research-proven health benefits of being active:

- Lower risk of vascular disease and heart disease.
- Longer life span and health during later years.
- Lower risk of heart attack and/or stroke
- Lower risk of high blood pressure or hypertension.
- Lower risk of high cholesterol.
- Lower risk of Type 2 Diabetes pre-diabetes or insulin resistance.
- Lower risk of bladder, breast, colon, esophagus, pelvic, kidney, lung and stomach cancers.
- Improved mental health, energy level and mood.
- Lower risk of dementia and Alzheimer's disease
- Improved overall quality of life.
- Reduced anxiety and depression.
- Improved sleep.
- Improved weight loss and reduced weight gain.
- Improved chance of keeping weight off.
- Stronger bones.
- Improved sexual function.
- Improved physical function.
- Improved flexibility.
- Improved strength.
- Lower risk of falls and broken bones in older adults.

Health benefits of daily activity for kids:

- Improved bone health and weight status in ages 3-5 years old.
- Improved ability to think and likely social, emotional and mental function aged 6-13 years old.

Health benefits of activity for pregnant women:

- Reduced risk of weight gain.
- Reduced risk of gestational diabetes.
- Reduced postpartum depression.

This list was adapted from the 2018 Guidelines for Physical Activity.

Something as simple as adding some physical activity to your daily life can improve your life in nearly every way! If exercise or physical activity was a new medication hitting the market - it would be sold out! It might not come in the form of a pill, powder or liquid but your health care provider can provide you with something to take daily. It's called an activity prescription and should include 15-30 minutes of movement daily! Feel free to talk to your health care provider for specific recommendations based on your situation and medical conditions. Again, if this isn't convenient then walk to the corner and back.

Trust me; every single health care provider would love to discuss ways for you to get healthier and less sick because they won't have to work as hard trying to medicate your various medical conditions in a thankless and futile effort to counteract the effects of poor nutrition and living a sedentary lifestyle.

There is literally no better treatment you can give your body for at least twenty medical conditions than simple, daily activity. Consider all of the medications you are currently taking for your medical conditions. Wouldn't it be great if you didn't have to take pills, injections, and capsules all day? Wouldn't it be great not to be sick and suffer the rest of your life? The way out of this dilemma is to perform daily, low to non-impact activity such as walking, riding a bike, lap swimming or light weights. A combination of these activities is even better.

For example, think about the heartburn you have after you eat meals and then sit down after dinner; it would likely improve if you went for a walk after dinner. Or consider the heaviness of the fluid in your legs you have on a daily basis due to some medical conditions. Walking daily would likely help return the fluid back into your blood vessels and get it out of your legs, wouldn't that be nice? Think about the vitamin D you might be low on; instead of taking a supplement with who knows what in it, you could go outside in the sunshine for 20 minutes since your body can usually make the vitamin D it needs. Or consider your blood sugar that seems to be always elevated and requires oral medication and insulin injections. Wouldn't it be great if a daily walk could lower your blood sugars and reduce the amount of medications you need to take? Well, it can and will, but you have to do it. And in order to do it, make it easy and you'll have much better success.

I can't promise any specific results, but most of the patients I work with who adopt these simple nutrition and activity habits, generally decrease their daily medication regimen, which is pretty cool. Each person's situation is different so talk to your health care provider and I can guarantee you can both agree on simple steps you can literally take to improve many medical conditions.

Physical activity is great at decreasing the levels in your body which are too high such as weight, blood pressure, cholesterol, blood sugar and is effective at increasing levels which are too low such as bone density, flexibility, mood and energy level.

Start Here to Get Active

There are hundreds of different ways to become more active. The goal is to start simple and get more complex over time if needed. I see a lot of people who sign up for intense workouts when they can't even walk around the block! They get injured or sore and end up discouraged. They lose motivation quickly and are back to square one. Find some activities you can easily add into your life such as walking, hiking, or pushups. Activity doesn't have to be heart exploding intense or cost anything. Just get moving!

> *"The journey of a thousand miles begins with one step."*
> ~Lao Tzu

This guide is designed to provide a new perspective and overall recommendation for increasing daily activity. This guide is intentionally not specific with routines or programs since everyone is in a different situation concerning their fitness level, medical conditions and past injuries. I recommend starting simply by going for a walk, riding a bike, some stretching, and a simple pushup and sit-up program on a daily basis. If you're alive, you can start here. If not, you're too late, sorry. It doesn't take great complexity to get great results. Start small and slowly and soon enough you'll be going further than you ever imagined. There are great resources in this guide. Check them out and I think you'll find them useful, easy to use, and best of all – free!

Stretching

Stretching is an awesome way to improve flexibility and prevent injury. There are a million different stretching programs available for free online. Also, yoga stretches and poses are very helpful to improve flexibility and reduce injury. Search for a PDF version of one designed by a medical clinic or physical therapy office, print it, and hang it up where you will be finishing your walk, light weight program or bike ride. Only stretch AFTER you are active. Never stretch much before being active. Muscles, tendons, ligaments and joints are not as flexible when they are cold. They will warm up as you are active or exercising. Always remember the saying: **Warm Rubber Bands Stretch, Cold Rubber Bands Break.**

Walking

> *"Walking: the most ancient exercise*
> *and still the best modern exercise."*
> ~Carrie Latet

By far the most effective habit for weight loss and to improve your overall health is to go for a daily walk. The daily walk has been the game changer for my patients over the past decade. They have experienced a ridiculous amount of life-changing success when they start walking daily. The reason is simple: 99.9% of people can incorporate a 15-30 minute daily walk into their lives with little to no effort. A daily walk doesn't require you to buy an expensive gym membership, new exercise equipment, or the latest gear. You never hear the latest fad exercise programs or diets recommend a daily walk because it seems too easy and isn't "insider knowledge." The ironic thing is, it works!

The benefits are significant and if you start walking daily, you will experience a transformation in your health and quality of life. How can this be? It's because a brisk, daily walk gives you a good chunk of time to get away, relax, and enjoy some time to yourself. These days, having some time to yourself during the day is hard to find. Remember, the goal of any activity recommendations in this book is not to add yet another activity to your life but to get more value and benefit from the activities you already do.

Instead of committing to some expensive or complicated exercise regimen, just start going for a simple walk once a day. Take a family member or friend and go explore your neighborhood or community. Maybe make a habit that you can't have dinner or sit down to watch television or the computer until you've gone for your walk. Once you have done this for a month or so, this will become a habit and you'll look forward to it. At this point you will be able to decide what to do next. Do you go farther, faster, or maybe start lifting some weights? Do you decide to add some stairs or maybe riding a bike next time? It's really up to you but remember, you need to walk before you run! Be sure to get your heart rate pumping a bit, maybe even a slight sweat and you'll know you are working hard enough. If you aren't able to talk while you are being active, then you are working too hard and need to dial it back a bit.

Our lifestyles have changed over time reducing the amount of activity we are getting both at work and at play. How many neighborhoods do you drive through in your town and see kids everywhere on their bikes and outside playing? It's very rare and ultimately the research reveals this is becoming a serious issue in our society as children are much less active and the rates of obesity and Type 2 diabetes in kids as young as ten years old are growing rapidly.

Another benefit of being outside walking is the community-building and security aspects. For example, during my education I moved several times across the nation and every time I moved to a new area, I drove around looking at different neighborhoods to see if there were kids outside playing and riding bikes. Even though I was driving through unfamiliar communities, I instantly had a pretty good idea which neighborhoods would be safe to live in versus those not as safe. When home owners are out walking and visiting with each other and a bunch of kids are playing outside, it seems like a natural deterrent to trouble-makers in my opinion.

> *"Walking is the best possible exercise.*
> *Habituate yourself to walk very far."*
> ~Thomas Jefferson

Many patients I've had over the years are very busy parents, business owners, executives and are also involved in the community. However, they are still able to incorporate a daily walk into their lives. In fact, many indicate their daily walk has significantly improved careers, businesses, relationships and health since they had the advantage of having time to think, plan and brainstorm during their walks. Overall, there are two ways these successful people use a daily walk. The first use is to take a break from the day and think about the big decisions and directions they wish to take in their professional and personal lives. Often, coworkers or family members think they are going for walk for only their physical health however the walk is actually for their physical, mental, and emotional health as well. So they are getting healthier in many ways and taking guilt-free time for themselves.

The second way people use their walking time is to be productive during their walk. Advances in technology has allowed music, podcasts, audiobooks and visiting on the phone to happen with our mobile phones and earbuds. These days we can do all kinds of activities while being on the move. Many salespeople take the time to make phone calls to clients to follow up and attend to their needs. Others listen to audiobooks and podcasts or complete continuing education which allows them to stay up to date in their field. Another patient who is in sales will call old friends and past clients in her contact list.

She's able to reconnect with old friends and clients and get her walk in as well. Review your responsibilities in life and brainstorm tasks you can complete while walking or riding a bike. It's always a rewarding feeling to get out and go for a walk while also getting some other required tasks completed. If you have children, have them walk too or ride their bikes while you go for a walk. They'll learn this habit and look forward to it each day. Also, this can also be valuable family time away from distractions which we all need.

To start walking, just start walking. It sounds simple because it is. No need to buy a $99 walking program or a contraption. Just start walking daily. Walk down to the end of the block if that's all you can do at first. Slowly, over time, try and walk a bit further until you are comfortable walking much longer distances, just be smart and safe. Keep it simple and take a walk!

Running or Jogging

For some reason whenever people want to get in shape they start a running or jogging program. If a person is overweight or obese this is pretty much the worst thing they could possibly do. Running causes high impact forces and jarring to your joints and muscles which can cause inflammation, pain and soreness. A significant amount of force goes through your ankles, knees, and hips when a person runs. Add extra weight to this and it's a recipe for disaster. If you are overweight or considered obese I do not recommend running for you. If you aren't overweight or obese, only at the point you can walk a mile or two at a reasonably quick pace should you even consider running. There is essentially no significant difference or benefit in energy expended for a person who walks at a quick pace or someone who runs. Save yourself pain, injury and from quitting and don't run when you're starting out. You'll be glad you avoided it.

Push-ups and Sit-ups

An even easier way to get started is to make a routine to do push-ups and sit-ups every day. These two exercises can be completed anywhere at any time and do not require any equipment. Start by doing a couple push-ups and see you many you can do. Strive to do this several times daily and see how many you can do in a day! Try and do at least five of each exercise twice a day and soon it will be a habit which can make the difference in your upper body strength and core strength. If push-ups are tough, start in a kneeling position instead of stretching out to balance on your toes, this is a bit easier and can help prevent injury as you are starting out. You can find some fun push-up and sit-up programs free online which can help you stay consistent. There is also at least one free app for your phone and tablet which will remind you and keep count of your push-ups each day. Before long you'll be able to drop and give me twenty without even a sweat!

Treadmill or Stationary Bike Indoors

Having a treadmill or stationary bike in your home is incredibly helpful for getting your daily activity completed. If you have a treadmill or stationary bike but don't use it, now's the time! If you don't have one, you might be able to find an inexpensive, quality, used treadmill or stationary bike that someone is excited to get rid of! I recommend putting them in front of the television or computer in your home. This way, you can be active while watching your favorite TV show or movie! Better yet, feel free to binge watch several episodes in a row and you'll have a much longer walk or ride to help get in shape. Try and do about 5 minutes at first and see how that goes. Based on that experience, you'll be able to decide how much you want to do the next day. The goal is to increase the time you are riding every week so you see progress. I recommend buying an inexpensive dry erase white board calendar and putting it up on the wall next to the treadmill or stationary bike. Write down either the time, distance or both of these each day and you'll see these numbers increase over time! It's very rewarding.

Walking With Friends

Some people use their time while walking to improve their friendships and spend quality time with loved ones. Some neighbors get together at 6:30 pm every night to go for a walk around the neighborhood and have great conversations about their families and life, which builds community. Others I know from different departments at work meet to discuss their day and get their exercise together. Interestingly, the employees who get out of the office at lunchtime seem to be more effective and refreshed in the afternoon than those who stayed and tried to get extra work completed.

Walking For Meetings

Some of my colleagues will go for a walk during lunch or during their working hours of the day to discuss important work issues in private. By going for a walk, they are able to have a personal meeting while addressing issues they need to cover. This allows them to not be stuck in a stressful office environment and helps them get some fresh air and seems to help them think and discuss decisions. These days, many employers realize the importance of having their staff standing or walking instead of sitting at desks all day. A walking meeting with an agenda can be very useful and effective for staff.

Walking In Weather

"The Americans never walk.
In winter too cold and in summer too hot."
~J.B. Yeats

While going for a walk the most important issue is your safety. If it's sunny when you walk I recommend sunscreen and maybe taking your water bottle if the weather is warm or hot. If you live in a region with heavy rains or winters, please dress accordingly and be prepared for slick sidewalks and drivers who likely don't know how to drive in bad weather. Wear shoes or boots with traction if it's icy or there is snow on the ground. Keep your phone nearby and always know where you are. Reflective clothing or headlamps are great to let drivers and others know you're there. Never assume they see you walking or crossing the road. Always be proactive rather than reactive about your safety.

Walking the Mall

A great way to get out of the house for people who stay at home or for our older generations is to head to the local mall for their daily walk. Most malls love having walkers cruising around in front of their stores as it brings people into the mall which helps their business while allowing the walker to get their walk completed in a safe, temperature-controlled, well-lit building. It's a win-win and helps everyone. Check out your mall announcement board or ask around. There is likely a great group of folks you will meet and you might be able to get in some social time while being active.

Walking the Dog

*"If your dog is fat, you're
not getting enough exercise."*
~Unknown

Dog owners are one of the most common walkers in most neighborhoods and around apartment buildings. Taking the dog for a walk is a great way to incorporate activity in your day. The dog is able to be outside and get some exercise while the owner also gets these benefits. These days there are many more dog parks which allow dogs to be off their leash and play with other dogs. If one is nearby, walk to it and let your dog run! Just don't be that guy who puts your dog inside the fence at the dog park and sits in your car eating potato chips – EPIC FAIL.

Riding Your Bike

One of the most underutilized forms of transportation in America is the bicycle. As children we gladly road bikes everywhere and no one thought a thing about it. I can remember being gone for hours of the day on my bike with friends running free. As an adult, I still love riding my bike because of the sense of freedom it provides. Riding a bike as an adult is like being a kid again. It allows us to go where we want and enjoy the ride, not only the destination. It is also an excellent source of non-impact exercise which helps every body system.

As people drive by in their 6,000 pound SUV and they see me riding my bike to work or to the store, their looks seem to say, "Poor guy, he must be homeless and he can't afford a car or maybe he has too many DUI's and has to ride his bike now." It's ironic and makes me chuckle due to the irony. They think the bike riders are the ones who are losing out and sacrificing. However, the bike riders are out enjoying the weather, getting some exercise, having some time to themselves to relax and think while listening to music or podcasts. And they are spending no money for the ride.

Meanwhile, drivers are spending nearly $1 per mile in gas, insurance, maintenance, tires, registration fees and taxes not to mention the high costs of taking care of eventual diseases associated with being sedentary. So, if you're an average American, then you drive about 10,000 miles per year, which costs you about $10,000 per year out of your bank account! Yikes, think about that next time you ponder where all your money goes each month. By the time someone uses common sense to compare the advantages of riding your bike for short distance activities compared to driving a car I figure the joke is on the driver - they just don't know it yet. Bike commuting to work is one of the best activities I do for myself. It's a great way to start a morning, gets your blood pumping and your mind fired up and ready for the day! I have a hands-free cell phone holder on my handlebars so I can listen to the latest podcast or audiobook which gets automatically downloaded for free to my phone from the public library's free app.

We became much more sedentary when automobiles became main stream in the 1940-60's. We stopped walking and riding bikes for errands such as commuting, grocery shopping, and our waistlines now reflect this. Find your old bike, tune it up and hit the road. It's amazing what we miss out on driving our two ton SUV's around. Riding a bike helps you, the environment, and your checking account.

When starting to ride your bike again, be smart and wear a helmet. Ride a ways and see how you feel. Start small and work your way up. Obey traffic laws and assume drivers have no idea you're there - because they don't!

Similar to starting walking, getting started riding a bike is to simply start riding. If you don't have a bike, then borrow one at first so you don't have to buy one until you are sure riding a bike will be something you will actually do. There are awesome deals to be found online and your local classifieds, including Craigslist. Start by riding around your neighborhood or at a local park to get started biking. Many communities have trail systems and rails to trails areas for safe bike riding. There is a nationwide program that has converted old byways used for railroad tracks to trails by removing the tracks. These wind through amazingly scenic areas of our nation and are great to explore.

Weight a Minute

Lifting weights is an incredible way to improve strength, flexibility, and endurance. Lifting weights can be completed with equipment at home or in the gym. Free weights or resistance bands seem to be the best and least expensive option. Using free weights and bands will also help build balance and coordination in your muscles to hold up a weight or perform reps correctly. Weight lifting machines can be used if you already have a gym membership however it's not necessary. There are tons of resources online to help you with starting a basic weight lifting program. Again, I recommend finding a cheap set of dumbbells, barbells, or resistance bands on Craigslist or some other local used site. Don't buy new unless you absolutely have to. Simply go online and you can find awesome sites with tons of helpful information. Stay away from any website which charges you a fee to use it or is trying to sell you something.

Swimming

Lap swimming, water aerobics and aqua classes are probably the easiest on your body of any exercises. That doesn't mean they're easy, it just means they aren't as tough on your body. Movement in water is easier on your joints and back than land-based exercise. Lap swimming is a great way to get aerobic exercise without the jarring effects of the ground. Even though it does require access to a swimming pool, it doesn't require much else besides a swimsuit, goggles and a swim cap. Most fitness facilities with pools generally provide relatively inexpensive swim lessons and classes on how to swim if you need to learn or hone your skills. Water-based aerobics classes aren't just for grandmas anymore. Many wellness centers even offer sessions where yoga is performed on paddle boards. Don't rush out and pay for an expensive gym membership just to use the pool. If you already have a membership, that's great. But if not, keep your cash and just start with the other forms of activity for now.

CHAPTER 7

SAVE TIME!

Most of our lives consistent of work time, home time and leisure time. The most simple and effective way to lose weight and improve your health is to simply incorporate physical activity into your daily life. I recommend simply changing some habits in your daily life to simply the process instead of adding more expensive gym memberships, commutes to the gym, workout gear, expensive gym equipment or nutritional supplements. There are no benefits to adding more costs in time and money to your life since you are likely already busy enough. This is one of the leading causes of failure with new weight loss and exercise programs. The LAST thing our modern life needs is more responsibilities in a day!

So, how do you do this? It's easy and incredibly time saving. The easiest way to get active is to get moving while completing activities you are already doing. This method is so effective; you'll wonder why you didn't do it years ago. The goal is to add motion to your regular daily activities. Sure, we've all heard the recommendations of parking further away from the store and taking stairs when possible. These are great ways to add some motion however they don't even scratch the surface of how easy it is to incorporate activity.

"Don't let the fear of the time it will take to accomplish something stand in the way of your doing it.
The time will pass anyway; we might as well put that passing time to the best possible use."
~Earl Nightingale

A word of caution: if there is no way you are going to get up early and get some exercise or activity in before work or school for example, then do not plan your exercise for the morning. Changing one habit to then change another one generally results in an epic fail pretty much every time. Changing one habit is hard enough but then relying on another habit to also change at the same time is worthless. It's called habit stacking and can sabotage the best efforts and plans. Set yourself up for success and fit activity or exercise in when it will be the easiest on you and your responsibilities. Who said this had to be hard or that you have to sacrifice to get healthy or in shape? You don't, so get out of that mindset. Don't give up mornings with your spouse or children if you don't want to. Also, don't give up evenings if these are the more important times for you. By adding physical activity into regular life tasks you'll get more done without missing out on the good stuff in life.

The basic idea behind increasing your ability to add your daily activity or exercise to your day is to learn how to multitask. Multitasking is the ability to perform several tasks simultaneously in order to increase your efficiency and save time. From a mental perspective, the ability to truly multitask has been shown to really not be possible. When I speak of multitasking, I'm describing a situation where you can do one activity while doing something else which doesn't require the same type of focus or mental awareness. Many of our daily responsibilities involve time when we are physically sedentary or sitting and could actually be moving. There are hundreds of ways to incorporate activity into your day from walking at lunch, using a stationary bike while watching television, calling customers or clients while walking, listening to audiobooks and podcasts while lifting weights are just a few. Once you see a couple examples of the concepts, evaluate your own life and see if there are easy ways to add some movement.

Don't Just Sit There

The saying goes, "if you're sitting then you're dying." The more sedentary we are, the more dangerous it is to our health. Therefore, many employers are allowing their staff to use variable height desks which rise and lower depending on the height the employee prefers. This allows employees to stand and move at their desks which is healthier and usually allows for better posture than those who sit all day. Consider trying an elevated desk and standing all day to see if this will help you feel better and work easier. Some employers are even installing treadmills at the workstations to allow employees to go for a slow walk while they work. Get creative and you'll appreciate the results and effective use of time.

Working Out in the Morning

*"I have to exercise in the morning before
my brain figures out what I'm doing."*
~Marsha Doble

If you are able to work out in the morning, then starting your day off being ahead of the game is a skill that can yield much higher results than you could ever imagine. If possible, change your schedule so you can exercise first thing in the morning before work or school. This may be tough at first, but most studies show that it takes about 21 days to create a new habit. If you can stick to it for that long, getting up early will become second nature.

My advice is to get up early on the weekend days too so you aren't constantly switching your schedule while trying to adopt the habit. If for whatever reason, you absolutely can't workout before work or get up early in the morning, don't stress about it. Once the habit is stuck, you'll be able to get some extra sleep on the weekends but still be able to get up early on weekdays. That way, you will have much more time off on during the weekend days to enjoy family and friends and get out and play instead of wasting the day sleeping!

By simply working out in the morning before work and family duties begin for the day, you have no way to miss your day's workout. It's done before you are barely awake and now you don't have to try and fit it in during your busy day. So when it comes to a busy work day, family responsibilities and last minute life disasters, you have no stress or guilt about not getting your workout in since it's already completed. Early morning workouts allow you to get your exercise in before the rest of the world is even functioning. While others are wasting time sleeping in, you are up and checking tasks off your list.

You may have coworkers that arrive at work and get more done in the first hour of their workday than everyone else in the office combined! Most everyone else is still working on getting another cup of coffee and trying to remember where their desk is! Most often these folks are early risers who have already been active or exercised before arriving to work. The "secret" is physical activity or exercise pumps oxygen-rich blood to your brain and helps you awaken and become alert faster. By getting to work in a ready-to-go state, you will have a more productive workday, guaranteed. Unlike your tired coworkers, you'll arrive and be ready to get some work done!

Social Time

Making your activity or exercise time a social time is a great way to spend quality time with friends and family while reaching your weight loss goals, perhaps together! Finding someone to exercise with is a great motivator for many people. Many participants will meet someone at the gym at a certain time. By having to be accountable to someone else, this increases the chance that you will stay committed to your physical activity program. Just make sure your workout partner doesn't end up talking you out of meeting at the gym or missing workouts. It's fine if they are going to miss a workout but that doesn't mean you should, too. Even better is finding someone that has the same goal as you do and creating workouts that meet both of your goals. Perhaps warming up on a treadmill or elliptical while visiting followed by a session of free weights while encouraging each other for that little extra effort will help strengthen your relationship and create a bond you can share. I encourage you to get out of the gym or your home and go for a walk or take a hike to explore the world around you! This will keep physical activity or exercise fun and interesting! By having someone else to go on an adventure with, you are creating memories, being safe and being active!

Lunchtime

The time set aside for lunch during our normal workday can be an enormous advantage if used correctly. How do you spend your lunchtime currently? Do you surf the internet, respond to random emails and pretend you are using the time wisely? Most of us waste this time in our day and have little to show for it. I remember reading a weight lifting book by Arnold Schwarzenegger in college. In the book, he discussed his ability incorporate more weight training into his week than most of his competition. He said the way he did this was simple. He realized that eating lunch really only took about 15 minutes out of the hour of time he was allotted for lunch. Once he was done eating, this left him around 45 minutes to get another session of weight lifting into his day! By doing this during the week, this added nearly 4 hours to his exercise total for the week and gave him a huge advantage over his competitors! This trick can easily be incorporated into any of our lives as well. It is very likely that right now as you read this you are thinking of about twenty excuses why you can't be active at lunch - 95% of these are excuses are complete crap. You know it and I know it. How many of us could use an energy pick-me-up for the afternoon that doesn't involve expensive coffees or energy drinks? When I'm active or work out during lunch, I am far more effective and productive in the afternoons. This is another secret trick to be a more productive employee whether you work for the boss or for yourself!

Simple ways to get active at lunch include:

• Using exercise facilities in your building provided by your employer.

• Seeing if a fitness center near your work has a discount for employees of your company. Sometimes they will give you a group discount if you and some colleagues join together - it doesn't hurt to ask!

• Changing your shoes and going for a simple walk while eating your lunch - simple sandwiches, string cheese, fruit, or granola bars are easy foods to eat on the move!

• Bringing your running/jogging clothes and getting your workout in during lunch.

After Work

Getting some activity in right after work is a great way to avoid a separate trip and save time. If you pass your fitness center on the way home, it's a great way to end your workday and blow off some of the stress you may have acquired throughout the day. I've always found the 5-7 pm time at the gym to be full of fun, social, and energetic people looking to start their evening off right. Of course, your main goal is to get your activity or workout in however it doesn't hurt to be occasionally social as long as you don't interrupt someone else's focus! Who knows, maybe you'll meet a new workout partner!

Wasted Evenings

I believe the evening hours are the most wasted time in our society today and here's why. Many people stay awake late into the evening to be entertained by the news or late night talk show hosts. Why? Generally it's a habit that we started before the days of internet and online video sources. Think about it, how many nights have you stayed up to watch the local news only to realize you already know most of the day's headlines? The daily news is easily accessible on any computer, cell phone, or tablet throughout the entire day and can be reviewed faster than any news anchor can read it to you. Why wait until late night to find out the day's news? One of the ways that many successful people I know keep up on current events is that they watch the news while they are exercising at home or at the gym. Most gyms have treadmills and elliptical machines strategically placed right in front of TV's so you can be busy being active and reaching your goals while not slowing your life down to read the freaking newspaper.

Late night talk shows are another example of an enormous waste of time at night. I truly have nothing against late night talk shows. They often have great interviews, "live" music and a hilarious take on news headlines. But, why stay up until almost midnight to watch these shows? If you can get to get to bed by 9 or 10 pm, you will almost automatically get enough sleep to get up a little earlier and start the following day ahead of the game. Now that we have streaming television, movies and YouTube, the old habit of staying up late to watch television shows should be extinct. Think about it, now you have the ability to enjoy media whenever and wherever you want. Also, I've found that there are tons of great podcasts that I can download and listen to while keeping up with the world, learning something new, and being active - all at the same time! This is an example of living life on YOUR schedule and terms, not on someone else's.

Some people can exercise in the morning however I've always had to work in the early morning hours so I would have had to wake up at 4am which didn't work for me. I literally trained for two Ironman triathlons and never once exercised in the morning. All of my workouts were during lunch or in the evening. Actually, over 80% of my training workouts occurred in the evening simply because I generally had to be to work by 7 am and the evenings allowed me a block of 1-3 hours for the various training sessions I needed to complete. I would often be swimming two miles worth of laps in the pool and not see another person! The most common excuse I hear about not exercising in the evenings is it can be hard to fall asleep after just exercising. I find most of this is unfounded and really isn't an issue once you get into a routine. In fact, crawling into bed within an hour or two of spinning for three hours is a welcomed option!

If you enjoy watching television or movies in the evening, put your treadmill or stationary bike in front of the TV. There is no reason why you can't be walking or riding at the same time. If you walked/ran/rode for an hour per night while watching your favorite shows, you would complete the entire amount of exercise required each seven days in just 4-5 days! It's a great time saver!

I care for a patient who is no longer Type 2 diabetic because she only allows herself to watch TV if she is riding her spin bike. She has significantly improved her health and not missed a moment of her favorite shows while doing so. She simply linked the habit of being active to a habit she really enjoys like watching her show and the result is remarkable! Who said you have to sit there in a vegetative state while watching your shows?

Weekend Mornings

Many people completely waste weekend mornings either hungover from a social event the night before or they choose to be lazy and not get much done before noon. After a long week of working, it seems natural to want to be a bit lazy on the weekends but don't let your workweek mess up your weekends too. Your weekday mornings are already spent getting ready and getting to work, why would you waste your weekend mornings too? One of the best times to get some great activity or exercise completed is to get up on a weekend morning and go find a fun physical activity such as a hike, bike ride, or swim! While everyone else is still getting motivated you can get some exercise in and also get your fun weekend started off right with something checked off your list and tons of energy left to enjoy your free time.

CHAPTER 8

SAVE MONEY!

One of the most debated aspects of losing weight and getting healthier is the perceived cost. In my opinion and experience, both of these habit changes should actually SAVE you money. It's true. By removing much of the processed foods which are all expensive and replacing them with whole, natural foods, you will save money. Also, not wasting money on expensive memberships or equipment will reduce the cost of changing your unhealthy habits. The following tips and tricks are designed to get you thinking about creative ways you can save money by reaching your fitness goals.

Another way being active and eating smarter is financially intelligent is to potentially decrease the cost of your health care when you are older. Saving for your retirement years is challenging enough but is made even more challenging when you have several chronic medical conditions and lots of expensive prescription medications since you didn't take care of your health during your working years. Most likely health care will continue to get more and more expensive as time goes on. It seems like a good idea to make an effort to reduce potential medical costs in the future if possible.

Fitness on the Cheap

Money is at the forefront of our minds these days, especially with the state of the nation's economy and our personal economy. Our society has been programmed to believe if you want to change something, you need to buy something. That is simply wrong. For a successful weight loss and get healthier program it is simply NOT necessary to buy a roomful of expensive equipment. If you can't currently complete twenty pushups and twenty pull ups at one time then you don't need a bunch of expensive weights. Treadmills can cost several thousand dollars while weight stations can cost three to four thousand dollars!

We are constantly bombarded with expensive new products on late night infomercials advertising if you pay ten easy payments of a hundred dollars, you will reach your weight loss goal! No doubt, you may actually use that piece of equipment dutifully for about a week and then clothes hangers start accumulating. Then "stuff" starts collecting on it, burying it under a pile of clutter. Congratulations, you just bought an overpriced closet rod and junk collector! When you buy expensive "stuff" to reach your goal, you are essentially hiring and employing the "stuff" to do all of the work for you instead of empowering yourself to do it. How many of us have said "that was expensive enough, I'd better use it" or "if buy this nice set of weights and videos, it'll force me to work out." The problem is we never use it. But "weight," there's more! Get it? Yep, that just happened.

When first starting out an activity program, the goal is to start simply and with the lowest cost possible. As far as I'm aware, I've never seen definitive research to prove that a person has better compliance over the long term after spending a large sum of money on a workout program or equipment than they do if they spend little to nothing.

Similar to a brand new car and truck, workout equipment such as treadmills, elliptical machines and weight machines lose much of their value the moment you purchase them. Simply look at ads on online classifieds and many times you'll see "Essentially brand new treadmill, used about 10 times, bought new last year for $1200, yours for $500, my loss your gain." If you've ever looked at classifieds you've seen an ad exactly like this one. So, if you can get a used but essentially brand new treadmill for over 50% off, why would you ever buy brand new equipment? It doesn't make sense. None of your uppity neighbors or in-laws really care about the newness of your gym equipment and if they do then they likely have bigger problems than you. By buying a used piece of equipment, you could easily save hundreds or thousands of dollars, dollars that could be spent on healthy food, family time, or put into your savings account.

The best places I've ever found to buy workout equipment are Craigslist, garage sales, thrift stores, and friends/family. Most people love it when you take used equipment off of their hands for a couple dollars. I once found a full weight set, barbell, dumbbells and a bench for $35. I still use this set to this day, I've had it for about 9 years. The set was at least $300 new, but I didn't pay it! I saved almost 90% off by purchasing used equipment in nearly new condition! Also, from an environmental standpoint, buying used equipment that would have otherwise ended up in the landfill is a great way to recycle. I'm not a landfill expert, but I suspect free weights and treadmills don't decompose very quickly. Since the equipment cost me so little to buy it doesn't give me a guilty feeling and I actually get a good feeling knowing it didn't end up in a landfill and it's still getting used daily. Be lean and green!

No Commute Necessary

Another huge time saver is having low cost exercise equipment at home instead of having to drive to the gym. By having the ability to be active at home, you essentially eliminate many different reasons most people won't get active.

Working out at home is a huge time-saver. No longer do you have to factor in driving time, costs of transportation, no transportation, and weather. Plus you save money by not paying for a gym membership. If you feel like you must have a gym membership, then that is perfectly fine. But, most people don't need to have access to a gym to get a great workout completed.

In order to get to the gym for me, it would take me about 20 minutes to drive EACH way. That means I have used 40 minutes of my day to workout and I haven't even been active or exercised yet during that time. If I factor in an hour workout then that's an hour and forty minutes I actually spent to work out! As you can see, by working out at home, you save yourself an incredible amount of time over months and years and will have an extra forty minutes in your day to do something else that needs to be completed like spend time with your kids, spouse, or have an extra cup of coffee. Also, in many areas of the country, winter is an imposing fact of life. When there is snow and ice on the ground, my travel time to the gym is longer and frankly, sometimes I don't want to leave a warm home to trek to the gym!

Being active at home is also a private way to workout. By working out at home you don't have to worry about other people in the gym as this can be intimidating and uncomfortable. You can stream workouts and online programs in the privacy of your own home and get the workout you need. This saves you from needing to spend a small fortune on dedicated workout clothes and shoes as well. Yeah, that old, torn t-shirt will work just fine if it's only you in your home. This helps by giving you the control of your environment so uncontrollable factors don't prevent you from getting your workout completed. Let's be honest, if the creeper or the grunter is at the gym at the same time as you, you're not going to get much of a work out completed.

Avoid Costly Memberships

Another cost barrier to starting a new activity plan is the cost of a membership to a gym, club, or fitness facility. One of the most frustrating experiences of my life was spent speaking with a "membership coordinator" at a trendy fitness club. They started out our conversation with these teaser rates and low monthly rates which all sounded great but when it came time to sign on the dotted line, the one-time "Initiation Fee" and "Administrative Fee" had added on about $300 to the cost to join. That amount spread out over the first twelve months of dues would have added $23 to my monthly teaser rate which effectively increased my monthly cost by 33%! I was furious! I know several business owners who own fitness facilities. They bank on only having a small minority of their members actually use their facilities. They realize most members will rarely, if ever, come in to the gym. How many months or years have you paid for gym membership and never even went! I know I have and I'm not alone.

Ultimately, I ended up joining the local YMCA which was a great experience. They electronically withdrew my monthly dues out of my checking account on a month to month basis with no long-term contracts. And, they also have minimal start-up fees. Another great fact about your local YMCA or community facility is that they generally have a fee scale based on your income and number of children. This makes it much less expensive for parents, especially in low income situations, to help themselves and also help their children start good activity and fitness habits early in their lives. The money I saved by joining the local, community gym was used to buy my entire set of home exercise equipment which my entire family can use anytime for the next several decades, and it's all paid for!

CHAPTER 9

SCHOOL IS IN SESSION!

It's important to get young or older students active to help develop these healthy habits so they can enjoy lifelong health and wellness. If you are a student you can significantly benefit from several smart habits whether you are in your early years, college years or maybe headed back for more education. In any of these scenarios you'll be better off if you can be learning while getting your daily activity completed. Avoid guilt while exercising by getting some school work completed at the same time.

Being a student is stressful and it seems like the first habit to go when school gets busy is your daily activity or exercise. Remember, it's guaranteed you'll get better results if you take care of yourself and studying while exercising is a great way to do this. And, exercise is a proven way to decrease stress, clear your mind and organize your thoughts. If you are sitting in the library for five hours every night drinking sugary soda to stay awake and feeling completely worn out, it's because you aren't taking care of your health and you're sabotaging your success. I know because I did this during my undergraduate days and it made school much more difficult than it had to be. In graduate school I focused on getting my exercise in and the difference in my energy level, focus and grades was truly shocking. Make it a point this semester to continue with your daily physical activity or exercise and you'll notice an enormous improvement in grades, sleep, quality of life, less depression and anxiety and you'll simply feel better.

Sure, some people go for a walk or to the gym to escape school work for a while; I get it. However, you probably also go out to parties, bars, play video games and watch movies over and over to avoid studying. You might as well retain the habit of being active or exercising while also getting your studying done since there is no way you're going to take your notes with you while you demolish others in a first person shooter video game with your friends!

Recording and Listening to Notes

One of the best ways to learn faster is to multitask using technology we already carry on us 24 hours per day. When I was in graduate school back in the day, I used to read many of my notes or outlines into a pocket voice recorder app on my phone and listen to my notes using headphones or earbuds while I ran outside or in the gym. Sometimes I would listen to my notes while riding my bike to class however traffic always seemed busy enough that I felt I needed to pay more attention and not daydream while studying.

The great part about this system is you are reviewing the information in multiple formats. You listen to the lecture and likely write or type notes, then you say the notes aloud into the voice recorder app on your phone, then you play it back and hear the information in your own voice and can emphasize certain points if necessary. By reviewing information this way, I can pretty much guarantee your information absorption rate will increase. It's a fact that physical activity and exercise oxygenates your brain and allows for better brain function. What better time to have increased brain function than while studying for your next exam? Instead of listening to the same music over and over, record your notes and go for a walk, run or bike ride and you'll be amazed and how much further ahead you are in your school work!

Memorizing Terms while Lifting Weights

Another trick I used when in school was making flash cards and looking at them in between workouts while weight lifting. I would read the card while in between sets and think about it while completing a set of reps. Once completed, I would move on to the next card and memorize this term while completing the next set. This method is great for memorizing keywords, terms, history dates and any other boring list of info you need to master. This is also a great way to learn another language. Most language learning systems are broken down into small sets of sounds and words which are perfect to practice while being active!

Studying on Stationary Equipment

It doesn't matter if you prefer paper or electronic versions of notebooks or tablets for learning. Both versions are incredibly useful to use while being active or exercising. These are easily placed onto treadmills, elliptical machines and stationary bikes to allow you to get your workout in while not feeling like you are going to get behind in your coursework. Also, for those who record lectures or their notes as previously mentioned, these files can be stored on electronic tablets and be played back using headphones or earbuds while in the gym or on an evening walk

Activity Summary

I recommend focusing on becoming more active each day with simple, low cost methods including walking, riding a bike and simple exercises like pushups and sit-ups. The most important aspect is finding what works for you and sticking with it on a daily basis. Being consistent is the most important part of incorporating a new habit into your life. Start simple with a specific daily activity and work your way up. Your body will tell you when it is time to increase your distance, pace, or time spent. Starting an intense fitness routine/program/club when you are very out of shape, overweight or obese will often result in injury, disappointment, and regret. I treat patients all the time who started an intense program designed for individuals who already have a basic level of fitness and have ended up injured since they didn't have any level of fitness. Start simple as this has proven time and time again to be the best starting point and foundation for becoming more active and developing healthy habits which will change the course of your life and health.

Find a simple activity such as going for an evening walk, bike ride or walk during lunchtime and you'll start a habit which will yield higher rewards than you could ever imagine! There is no need to empty your bank account and fill up your calendar with expensive, time-sucking exercise programs. Consistency is the key and the formation of a daily activity habit will provide this for you.

This is the secret you've been looking for and fortunately it's completely free and you can start NOW!

FUNDAMENTAL PRINCIPLES

• Change a couple basic habits and you'll basically save your own life.

• Eating healthier and getting more active is NOT more expensive. In fact, you will SAVE money!

• If something is easy or convenient, consider the cost you are paying with your health, weight, or bank account. For example, your overweight neighbor who pays some thin guy to mow his lawn. Classic.

• Time should NEVER be a barrier to being active or consuming healthier food. We only get so many days so enjoy being and feeling healthy with lots of energy and having fun.

• Nutrition Rule: Don't eat it if it hasn't lived before or is in cardboard, plastic or an aluminum can.

• Never buy products advertised as Low Fat, Reduced Fat, Lite, Fat Free, etc. They're all expensive chemical bombs!

• NEVER buy expensive workout equipment, memberships, expensive supplements, or workout programs to lose weight.

• Losing weight, maintaining weight, or gaining weight all require specific habits that when used, provide the intended results.

• Counting calories is stupid. Do it if you want but once you eat healthier foods, lower your carb intake, and start a daily walk - it all works out.

• NEVER restrict any food from yourself. Make the time for your family or friends and enjoy their birthday cake if you want. Life is short. If you indulge in a treat, enjoy it, and then get back to your plan. Life is a marathon, not a sprint.

• If it's found in the store's bakery, its garbage. Especially whole grain. Carbs like breads, pastas, grains, potatoes are garbage. Seriously, avoid them.

• Don't get hung up on details and specifics - results happen when you're consistent daily with the basics.

REFERENCES AND RESOURCES

This guide refers to various sources of research and publications provided by the Centers for Disease Control and studies produced by our government. This publicly available information is incredibly thorough and accurate. It is available free online and is the hub for medical providers and the public as well. I didn't have to research and locate specific facts and statistics for this guide since I use this commonly known data on a daily basis. However, I believe it is very important to provide you with all the sources necessary to verify information presented here as well as give you a starting point to look into these topics more in depth for your own knowledge and benefit. Below are links in several key areas which are incredibly valuable for you to have. Best of all, they are all free.

The United States government has spent an enormous amount of your taxpayer money to research, evaluate, and create incredible guidelines and resources for US citizens as well as anyone else worldwide who can benefit from the information. I intentionally did not provide specific work out programs, images of exercises or tables in an effort to keep this guide as inexpensive and efficient as possible. Therefore, use these links to find more information or guidance concerning any topic presented in this guide. **It's free and yours to use!**

General Statistics, Fast Stats and Trends
• www.cdc.gov. 2018. Data and Statistics.[ONLINE] Available at: https://www.cdc.gov/obesity/data/index.html. [Accessed 1 December 2018].

• NHANES. 2018. National Health and Nutrition Examination Survey. [ONLINE] Available at: https://www.cdc.gov/nchs/nhanes/index.htm. [Accessed 1 December 2018].a large amount of great data and results.

2018 Guidelines for Physical Activity
• www.health.gov. 2018. Current Guidelines. [ONLINE] Available at: https://health.gov/paguidelines/second-edition/. [Accessed 1 December 2018].

Overweight and Obesity Info
• www.cdc.gov. 2018. Overweight and Obesity. [ONLINE] Available at: https://www.cdc.gov/obesity/index.html. [Accessed 1 December 2018].

Type 2 Diabetes Info
•www.cdc.gov. 2018. Type 2 Diabetes. [ONLINE] Available at: https://www.cdc.gov/diabetes/basics/type2.html. [Accessed 1 December 2018].

ABOUT THE AUTHOR

Eric J. Belanger, PA-C, MPAS, has been a physician assistant for eleven years in orthopedic surgery and pain management. Born and raised in Montana, his early years were spent exploring high mountain lakes in the Beartooth Mountains with a backpack and a fly rod. College years took him to Bozeman, Montana to explore trout streams and biomedical research labs. After graduate school in Idaho, he worked for six years in Spokane, Washington where he was lucky enough to meet his wife Elisha and also creatively found some time to complete two Ironman triathlons and a bunch of other endurance races. In 2012, they moved to the Flathead Valley in Montana to raise their two sons, Ben and Nate, with as much wilderness nearby as possible. In his free time outside of the medical field, he enjoys camping, boating, skiing, fishing and being outdoors as much as possible.

Made in the USA
Columbia, SC
24 December 2019